RECALL
ABORTION

RECALL ABORTION

Ending the Abortion Industry's
Exploitation of Women

Janet Morana

Foreword by Fr. Frank Pavone
Introduction by Teresa Tomeo

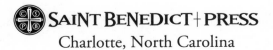

SAINT BENEDICT + PRESS
Charlotte, North Carolina

Cover design by Caroline Kiser.

Cataloging-in-Publication data on file with the Library of Congress

ISBN: 978-1-61890-960-2

Published in the United States by
Saint Benedict Press, LLC
PO Box 410487
Charlotte, NC 28241
www.saintbenedictpress.com

Printed and bound in the United States of America

More praise for *Recall Abortion* . . .

Janet has captured the reality of abortion from the woman's perspective—a view that has been missing in the abortion debate. We discuss a woman's right to have an abortion but, until *Recall Abortion* no one followed up to see what impact that right has had.

> —Georgette Forney, President Anglicans
> for Life, Co-founder of the Silent
> No More Awareness Campaign

Janet Morana delves into the many reasons why abortion should indeed be recalled. Her book enables you, the reader, to come along side Janet as she explores various aspects of so-called "reproductive choice." In the process, she negates the arguments by pro-abortion activists. As a long-time veteran of the pro-life movement, she's got a lot to say.

> —Bradley Mattes, President, International
> Right to Life Federation

I've known Janet Morana for a long time, and I know her to be a passionate and effective advocate for America's unborn babies and their mothers. I highly recommend her book as a helpful tool to counter the rhetoric of radical pro-abortion activists.

> —J.C. Willke, MD, President, Life
> Issues Institute

Recall Abortion will help put abortion right where it belongs; on a worldwide "Hall of Shame" episode and the top of the recall list.

> —Teresa Tomeo, Syndicated Catholic
> Talk Show Host, Best-Selling
> Catholic Author

In *Recall Abortion*, Janet Morana intertwines her personal experience with the powerful, riveting stories of other women and families caught in the lies and painful consequences of the "sexual revolution" of the twentieth century. Documenting the tragic effects, over decades, of abortifacients and abortions, Janet convincingly demonstrates that we neither need nor want abortion, even in the "hard cases" of rape and incest, fetal anomalies, or "life of the mother." We can do better!

—Margaret H. Hartshorn, Ph.D.,
President; Heartbeat International

In this book Janet took a risk and told the truth about abortion—*Recall Abortion* is a masterpiece.

—Mother John Marie Stewart, Founder,
Disciples of The Lord Jesus Christ

After 40 years on the market, has abortion lived up to its promises? *Recall Abortion* provides a compelling case against the primary selling points for abortion."

—Wendy Wright, Former President and
CEO, Concerned Women for America
Current position: Vice President for
Government Relations and Communications for the Catholic Family and
Human Rights Institute (C-FAM)

To my daughters, Jennifer, TaraLynn, and Kelly:
You taught me that life is the most precious gift—
You're the inspiration for everything I do.

CONTENTS

abortion is simply between Republicans and Democrats;

others think it is between religious and non-religious people, or between conservatives and liberals.

In the end, this book calls for a brand new dividing line: between those who really care about the people who have abortions, and those who don't care, between those for whom caring trumps ideology and those whose ideology causes them not to care, between those who are willing to listen and those who have lost the ability or will to do so.

That dividing line, it seems to me, offers the best hope of solving the abortion crisis in our nation and in the world.

FATHER FRANK PAVONE
National Director,
Priests for Life

INTRODUCTION

A S SOMEONE who worked as a general assign-
ment reporter for more than twenty years in radio
and television, I covered many stories involving product
recalls. Recalls in the auto industry, for example, were
semi-regular news items in my hometown of Detroit.
The car companies would issue a press release on Friday
afternoons, hoping that newsrooms winding down for
the weekend wouldn't pay much attention. But at least
they were, for the most part, forthcoming with the basic
information. It was a matter of customer satisfaction and,
of course, liability. If they weren't upfront they would pay
for it either in decreased sales or lawsuits or in some cases
both. That's because the car companies and other major
product and service providers know that Americans are
savvy consumers. In addition to possible boycotts or legal
action, today's customers have many ways to voice their
concerns, and those ways go well beyond alleging false
advertising or filing complaints with the Better Business
Bureau.

Most media outlets devote a good amount of air-
time or copy to consumer complaints. They're attention
grabbers; the things that ratings, headlines, and newspaper sales are made of. After all, just about everyone at

some point in their life has had an experience of being an unhappy customer. In Detroit, one network affiliate is known for its "in your face" approach to con-artists with weekly "Hall of Shame" segments. The reporter, responding to a letter or email from a viewer, chases down the crooked contractor, and shames him or her into fessing up and paying up. There are countless magazines, newspaper articles, and web sites devoted to advice for the savvy shopper. And in addition to professional rip-off artists being exposed by a vast variety of news media, the issue of spending money wisely has morphed into many popular TV reality shows. Whether it's cars, coupons, or the perfect little cottage or villa on Lake Cuomo that's for sale, by golly we are going to get what we were promised. And the media are right there with us ready for lights, camera, and action—*except* when it comes to one of the biggest rip-offs of all time: abortion.

That is why this powerful book by my dear friend and Catholic media colleague Janet Morana is so important. The world has been sold a huge bill of goods when it comes to the billion dollar business of abortion. It affects more than the innocent baby in the womb. It affects more than the woman undergoing the heinous procedure. It affects more than the father of the child, who is often left out of the "choosing." Abortion continues to take a huge toll on society in so many ways. As Janet documents so precisely, abortion has not lived up to any of its promises. In addition to taking the lives of thousands of human beings every day around the globe, those who provide abortions have engaged in one of the most influential and fraudulent scams in the history of God's green earth.

I used to consider myself pro-choice. Believe it or not, despite my years of experience as a journalist, I too believed the sales pitch of the abortion movement. It wasn't until I was assigned to report on welfare funded abortions in my home state of Michigan that my eyes slowly began to open. Back in the early 1980s when voters were being asked to end welfare funding, a wonderful pro-life nurse laid out a long list of facts for me concerning women who are pressured into abortions as well as the countless safety issues at abortion facilities. I was stunned. I was mad at myself for not using my skills to get the facts earlier. I was furious at my profession for not only going along for the ride but for aiding and abetting the abortion industry at every turn, and only doing the bare minimum when it came to reporting the other side of the story. And I was furious with the Planned Parenthoods and NARALs (now NARAL-Pro Choice America) of the world, who proudly and arrogantly proclaimed they were so concerned with reproductive health when abortion has absolutely *nothing* to do with either reproduction or health! In addition to keeping so many in the dark about the ugly realities of one of the most profitable scams going, these so called "women's groups" also blatantly ignore the cries of fellow women who learned the hard way that abortion is harmful. So much for sisterhood!

As someone who knows media and public relations, I can say that the abortion industry and its many partners in crime, including Planned Parenthood, NARAL-Pro

Choice America, political action committees, EMILY's List, and the countless politicians at the state and federal levels, all get big fat As for their marketing efforts. They have been so successful that abortion has become synonymous with women's health. It's called a "choice" and now even a "right." Anyone who publicly disagrees is considered out of touch and accused of wanting to hurt, not help, women.

But it is never too late. Fr. Frank Pavone of Priests for Life says we can only suppress the truth for so long. He has another great line which I use often in my talks and on my radio program when discussing the lies of the abortion industry: "You can't practice vice virtuously." Slowly but surely the truth about abortion is being revealed. *Recall Abortion* will help put abortion right where it belongs: on a worldwide "Hall of Shame" episode and at the top of the recall list.

TERESA TOMEO
Syndicated Catholic Talk Show Host
Best-Selling Catholic Author

CHAPTER ONE

A New Perspective on Life

WHEN I was an early childhood public school teacher in New York City, most of my colleagues considered themselves pro-choice. My good friend and team teacher Denise adamantly proclaimed her pro-choice views, while I was the token pro-lifer.

One spring we decided to hatch chickens in our classroom. We ordered all the appropriate equipment, including our precious fertilized eggs. The children were so excited to watch nature unfold right before their eyes.

One morning when we entered the classroom, Denise and I noticed a problem with one of the eggs. The shell was cracked and we could see a yellow yoke sac and a pulsing, bloody mass. It was the beating heart of a chick that was not going to develop further. Denise and I were both upset. Denise gasped, "It is still alive!" It was, but there was nothing we could do to save it. Within moments the chick's heart stopped beating. Denise was saddened by the loss of this chick in the very early stages of development.

How could Denise be pro-choice on abortion and yet feel such sadness at the loss of a pre-born chicken?

She was obviously a very sensitive person but when it came to unborn children, her logic seemed to vanish. This is not uncommon. Many people who consider themselves pro-choice think it is perfectly fine to terminate the life of an unborn child in the first trimester. So why is it that when it comes to animals, people are suddenly so pro-life?

Consider dogs. A pedigree pooch is pregnant with a litter of six puppies, while a mixed breed also is pregnant with a litter of six. The owner of the pedigree will have no problem selling those six puppies and making a decent profit. The owner of the mixed breed, on the other hand, will probably have a difficult time finding homes for the puppies. Why not abort the mixed-breed puppies? After all, aren't there enough stray dogs wandering the streets already? Well, you can bet if word got out there would be a public outcry and extensive media coverage. We don't tolerate aborting dogs, but aborting human children is considered a "right."

Why is it that when we talk about the destruction of human lives from abortion, our conversation is cloaked in terms like "a woman's right to choose," but with puppies, there is an almost unanimous pro-life opinion?

Consider for a moment the term "pro-choice." It sounds quite good. In fact, it is very American to support freedom of choice. But there are clearly instances when freedom of choice must be limited because it infringes on the rights of another person. For example, I do not have the freedom to choose to smash a car, steal from a store, or assault or kill another human being. Yet when it comes to abortion, we discuss the killing of an unborn child in the feel-good vocabulary of a woman's right to choose.

We have the right to choose many things—where we live, what kind of car to drive, where to send our kids to school—but the term "pro-choice" is used so loosely when it comes to abortion. Have we sufficiently considered what is being chosen, what an abortion is, and what consequences it has? Does the use of the word "choice" rather than the word "abortion" mask a deep discomfort we have with the reality of abortion, and an admission— at least deep within—that it is profoundly wrong?

Often the last thing supporters of legal abortion want to discuss is abortion. Furthermore, many Americans have no idea about the ins and outs of abortion or what the Supreme Court decision *Roe v. Wade* was about, because the issue of abortion isn't even on their radar screen. I know, because I was once like that. Let me tell you about my journey from being ambivalent on abortion to passionately pro-life.

While I never considered myself pro-choice I also wouldn't have labeled myself pro-life. The truth is, I never gave abortion a second thought while I was growing up in the 1960s and 1970s.

I was born in Brooklyn, New York, in 1952 and educated in Catholic schools. I am the oldest of four children, with fourteen years separating me from my youngest sibling. I grew up before the Second Vatican Council, and the Catholic Church and liturgy were very different from today. The Mass was in Latin, and the priest celebrated Mass with his back to the congregation. Women had to have their heads covered with either a hat or a chapel veil before entering the church. Everyone genuflected before entering the pew, and the tabernacle was in the center of the church. Our catechesis was from the Baltimore Catechism, which was written in a question-and-answer format.

Spiritual direction didn't exist for the average layperson. You memorized all your prayers, and you followed the Mass with your St. Joseph Missal. Just about every Saturday afternoon, kids would come in from playing to change clothes and walk over to church for Confession. On Sunday morning you lined up in the school yard for the 9 o'clock Children's Mass. Church was a place of warmth, comfort, and stability. In fact, when meeting new people, you commonly identified yourself by the name of your parish—mine was St. Vincent Ferrer, in the Flatbush section of Brooklyn. But you would just say, "I'm from St. Vinny's!"

The Second Vatican Council ended in 1965 and the Church of my childhood began to undergo some radical changes. The whole look of St. Vinny's began to change. The altar was turned around, the priest faced the congregation, and the Mass was now all in English. Latin hymns and organ music practically vanished, and in came the guitars, tambourines, and folk music. The tabernacle was dismissed to a side altar, the beautiful marble altar railing was removed, and we no longer knelt to receive communion; in fact, we were encouraged to receive Jesus in our hand. Confession could now take place face-to-face with the priest, and ours began to discourage weekly Confession anyway—a monthly or even "seasonal" confession was considered fine. Women no longer had to have their heads covered upon entering church. Genuflecting almost became passé. That feeling of awe at being in the presence of Christ when you entered the church had changed. Imagine being an adolescent going through this. The one sure, stable thing you thought you could count on was radically changing. This was a time that tried people's souls.

I attended high school at St. Agnes Seminary, a small, all-girl Catholic high school in Brooklyn, staffed by the Sisters of St. Joseph. In my sophomore year, 1968, the Church went through another radical change.

On July 25, 1968, Pope Paul VI issued his encyclical, *Humanae Vitae*. Many expected him to drop the Church's ban on artificial contraception, but he did just the opposite: he reaffirmed the Church's stance. The issue of contraception began to cause a divide in the Church. You could go to a priest on one side of a church and be told that birth control was a sin, while on the other side of the same church another priest would say it wasn't a sin as long as you had a "good reason."

Along with the growing divide within the Church, the culture outside of it was also changing. In came the sexual revolution, "women's liberation," and the drug culture. I have to confess that I got caught up in this changing world. I began to question my faith. I no longer believed in the infallibility of the pope. I thought women had a right to birth control. All those Baltimore Catechism questions and answers became irrelevant to me.

I distinctly remember the moment when I took my first step down the slippery slope away from the Church.

It was my sophomore year in high school, and the priest came to our school for our monthly Confession. I dutifully lined up with my class, but I began to feel anxious and no longer wanted to go to Confession. I did an about-face and walked back into class. Sister asked, "Confession, Janet?" and I lied, "Yes, Sister." It was my first step away from the Church that had nurtured me. I stopped going to Confession, which led me to abstain from Communion, which in turn led to me skipping Mass altogether. Before long, I only attended Mass on Christmas and Easter.

I remained aloof from the Church throughout high school and college. In 1974 I graduated from St. Francis College, and I got married a year later. My Catholic faith no longer mattered to me, and my relationship with God was almost non-existent. At the same time, all my close friends were getting married, so marriage just seemed like the next step to take.

I became engaged after dating my future husband for three months. From there things moved quickly towards our wedding day. At Pre-Cana classes, the priest told us that depending upon the circumstances, birth control pills could be an option for us. I didn't realize at the time that this was bad advice in every way—theologically, spiritually, psychologically, and physically.

As the oldest of four siblings, I had many years of experience changing diapers and babysitting, and felt that delaying the start of a family was a good idea. I had taken birth control pills back in high school (although I wasn't sexually active), as prescribed by my Catholic gynecologist for menstrual problems. With both a priest and a doctor legitimizing the use of contraceptives, I continued my journey down that slippery slope.

I started taking birth control pills three months before my wedding. About a month before our wedding, my fiancé began to pressure me sexually. I was a virgin but gave in to the pressure, and so my marriage got off to a bad start. When you begin marriage not knowing each other very well and compound things by moving into an intimate physical relationship, you set the stage for disaster. There's a popular song about marrying your best friend. That's how well you should know someone before entering into such a serious, lifelong commitment. Unfortunately, we didn't heed that advice.

I continued taking the Pill for two years. Once I stopped, I got pregnant immediately and gave birth to an absolutely beautiful baby girl, Jennifer. I threw all my attention into motherhood, and as a result I wanted to delay having another baby. I went back on birth control pills until my daughter was thirteen months old. I felt it was important for her to have a sibling, so I stopped taking the Pill. Once again, I became pregnant almost immediately. The (untrue) lesson I was teaching myself was this: no Pill equals countless children.

This time I gave birth to beautiful twin girls, Tara and Kelly. By this time, birth control pills were being linked with an increased risk of blood clots and strokes. With a history of strokes in my family, I was afraid to go back on the Pill, and I didn't know about Natural Family Planning. In fact, the only natural method I knew of was the old "rhythm" method, which was considered by most to be unreliable. Since my marriage was built on a physical relationship, you can imagine the fighting that began.

When the twins were three, I thought I was pregnant again. It was just a scare, but it was enough to make me do something really drastic: I had a tubal ligation. I thought all my problems were solved. I was wrong.

I had embraced everything the feminist movement promoted as being liberating and empowering for women. In reality, I had not been liberated; every day I felt more trapped in a bad marriage. As my marriage continued its downward spiral, I focused more and more on my three daughters. It was also around this time that I reconnected with my Catholic faith.

It is amazing how the hand of God works. I was trying to get a job teaching in the public schools on Staten Island, but not only were they not hiring, they were also instituting budget cuts. My mother-in-law, who was a daily communicant and who took my daughters to Mass every Sunday, began praying a novena that I would find a job. I just rolled my eyes, being the "Doubting Thomasina" that I was. But sure enough, two days before Christmas 1988, I was hired to teach first grade in P.S. 31 in Staten Island. It was a miracle!

My mother-in-law instructed me to go to church and light a candle of thanksgiving. Since it was Christmas and I went to Mass then anyway, I lit my candle. I made it to Mass again the following Sunday, not wanting to risk my good "luck" as I started my new teaching position.

I found myself at Mass for a third straight Sunday, and the hand of God reached out to me again. We were leaving church when my daughter Tara called out to the newly ordained Father Frank Pavone to come over and meet me. She said, "Father Frank, here's my Mom. You know, the one who needs to go to Confession!" I turned beet red with embarrassment.

Father Pavone was very cool and tempered Tara's excitement. He turned to me and told me I didn't have to go to Confession. Well, that was a relief! But he gave me the rectory phone number and told me to give him a call. He said we could just talk.

Just talk about the Church? That seemed odd to me. So I stuffed the paper with his number in my pocketbook and there it stayed for a few more weeks, until one day I stumbled across it again and decided to give the young priest a call. He invited me to his Friday night Bible class and we set an appointment for spiritual direction.

When we met, I gave him my laundry list of disagreements with the Church's teaching and he wasn't shocked. He invited me to continue with the Friday night Bible class, and I took him up on the challenge. After three months of discussion and study, I was finally ready for Confession. After twenty years away from the Church I rediscovered the wealth of our Faith. I received Communion that day, and it was just like my First Holy Communion. I knew I was beginning a relationship with Jesus.

As I continued to rediscover my faith and the teachings of the Church, I learned about God's beautiful plan for marriage, including Natural Family Planning. I also became aware of how birth control pills really worked.

I always thought they simply prevented fertilization.

But I learned that the Pill actually has its own built-in insurance policy, employing several different methods in case one or more don't work. Besides trying to prevent fertilization, the Pill also thickens the cervical mucus, which then acts as a barrier, preventing the sperm from getting to the egg. If both of these first two methods fail and ovulation and conception both occur, then the Pill acts to prevent the fertilized egg (the newly conceived human being) from implanting itself onto the side wall of the uterus. The child is then aborted out of the body.

I didn't feel the impact of this newfound information until several years later. I was with a friend visiting the Epcot Center in Disney World, and we decided to check out the Wonder of Life exhibit. As I watched a beautiful video showing the miracle of how life begins, I realized what taking the birth control pills really meant: *the possibility of aborting new life.* In the years that I had been taking birth control pills, I had been very sexually active. I also knew that I was an extremely fertile woman. Given these facts, I have no doubt that I had successfully conceived new life many times, but had never given those babies the chance to grow inside me. For the very first time in my life, I came to grips with the fact that I had not only shut myself off to life, but had also *destroyed an unknown number of children.*

As I came out of the exhibit, I walked over to a nearby fountain and began to sob uncontrollably. I stayed there for some time, washed in grief and remorse. For the first time, I was aware of the full impact of what I had done.

As I became involved in pro-life work, I learned more about the damage abortion does to women. I realized that many post-abortive women feel alone in their grief at first, and ashamed to express it, but later are able to experience mercy and healing. These women who had been through the healing process could therefore serve as a voice for other women still locked in the secret sin of abortion.

I recognized how important these women could be to the pro-life movement, so I co-founded the Silent No More Awareness Campaign, an initiative that gives women a forum for publicly testifying about the negative impact abortion had on their lives.

Because I never had a surgical abortion, some began to question why I was involved in such a campaign. Here again, I had to come to grips with all the children I had lost because of birth control pills. When working in post-abortion ministry, it's tempting to recognize only the pain and grief that comes from surgical abortion. Yet the loss I feel is just as real as if I had had a surgical abortion. Moreover, I know I am not alone. Many women have shared with me their grief from years of taking abortifacients.

I am now reaching out to others who share these feelings, and have found time and time again that I am not the only woman with a testimony like this. I know we can help many families realize the damage birth control can cause in their lives. I also want to reach out to others who feel the pain I have described and tell them that they, too, can take the first steps towards healing.

It is my hope that others like me who turned their back on Jesus and the Church will realize the true wealth we have in the documents and teachings of the Church, and the power the Lord gives us to live those teachings. It is my hope that they see their purpose in life is, as the Baltimore Catechism said, "To know, love and serve Him on Earth so that we may be happy with Him in Heaven." Ah! But now see that we are called to know Jesus Christ as our Lord and Savior and also as our friend. We are called to have a personal relationship with Him. I nearly threw this all away and was away from Him for almost twenty years. I will spend whatever time I have left here on earth singing His praises and hopefully, through my story, bringing others back to the Lord and His Bride, The Church!

So now you can see why I am so passionate about the life issue. At one time I was clueless but once I discovered the truth it was like an iron door closed behind me and I couldn't go back. Nor would I want to.

You now know how I made my journey back to the Catholic Church and into the pro-life movement but how and why did I think of recalling abortion?

In my years working in the pro-life movement, I have worked with many of the leaders in the movement, and I also have been in many strategy meetings. In 2002, while planning activities for the thirtieth memorial of the *Roe v. Wade* decision, I brought forth the idea that we needed better messaging with women. The voice of those who had experienced abortion was glaringly absent from the abortion discussion. Experience always trumps rhetoric. I co-founded the Silent No More Awareness Campaign to give a platform to those voices speaking out about the physical and psychological pain that abortion had brought to their lives. What we found was an outpouring of grief and regret; testimonies that spoke to the immense pain and suffering that abortion causes.

In 2011, we began to look ahead to January 22, 2013, when we would mark the sad day of forty years of legalized abortion in America. It was in those meetings that I got the idea of recalling abortion all together. There has been progress at the state level placing some limits on abortion. My idea is that abortion is not real medicine since it stops the body from doing what nature intended. In fact, it's the opposite of medicine, as it actually harms women. Any other product that had the massive negative effects that abortion does would be taken off the market!

Abortion is a bad product, plain and simple. Abortion is obviously a bad product for the babies because it kills them. But it is also a bad product for the mother because of the physical and psychological damage it causes. It's bad for the father and for the entire family. Yes, it is even bad for our society as a whole. As you read on you will see the evidence for taking the procedure off the market and demanding a government recall of the product called abortion.

CHAPTER TWO

WHY RECALL ABORTION?

A BORTION IS the greatest hoax ever perpetrated against women, and those who profit from abortion are the snake oil salesmen of our time. This statement may strike some as sensationalism, but I assure you it is not. The evidence presented in this book will show that it is no exaggeration.

Abortion is one of the most common surgical procedures performed on women in the United States and, statistically speaking, one-third of American women will have at least one by age forty-five. It is legal to have an abortion through all nine months of pregnancy, even for healthy babies and healthy mothers. Most abortions are performed in free-standing abortion clinics that operate virtually unregulated. In fact, many states have strict laws protecting your pets in veterinary clinics, while few laws protect women (or, certainly, babies) in abortion clinics. States that attempt to impose regulatory oversight on abortion invariably end up defending those rules in court.

Pro-aborts argue that the regulations restrict women's access to health care. But is abortion really health care? It's a statement that has become such a common refrain in political rhetoric that many just accept it as truth.

How many of us have truly thought about it in those terms? Most surgeries either correct something the body is doing wrong (like growing tumors) or help the body do something it is supposed to be doing but can't (like keeping organs functioning properly). Abortion, on the other hand, stops the body from doing what it was designed to do. A woman's body is uniquely designed to bear children, and to feed and nurture those children after they're born.

Let's compare abortion to other ambulatory surgeries. If you need to have, say, gallbladder surgery, you meet with the surgeon a few weeks before the surgery is scheduled. After the date is set, you typically go to the hospital the week before for pre-admission tests like a chest x-ray, urine analysis, and blood work. The day of the surgery, you arrive at the hospital, usually in the morning, and the intake nurse asks you a battery of questions. You meet with your doctor, again, and he or she asks the same questions, and some new ones. If you haven't already met with the anesthesiologist, you will that morning. Before administering any kind of sedation, the anesthesiologist will ensure that you have not eaten or had anything to drink. He will ask you how much you weigh, or if you have had any previous sensitivities to sedation drugs. Before you go under, the surgeon and anesthesiologist make sure you understand the procedure you are about to undergo, and what to expect as you recover.

After the procedure, the surgeon will come to see you in recovery, or meet with a family member in the waiting room to discuss how the surgery went. After a

nurse showed me into a room where I was supposed to change. But I couldn't change; I just sat there and cried. The nurse returned and quickly became angry as she saw me sitting there, still in my clothes. She told me to change and said "Do it NOW!" She left me there again to change. This time I did, and I cried the whole time. So much was running through my mind and I wanted to leave so badly. But I didn't.

As I was lying on the table, I felt humiliated. The doctor looked at me and said to the nurse "Oh, we'll see this one here again." I looked at him and said "you will never see me again." He laughed as he replied, "yeah, right, that's what they all say." I felt so alone and afraid.

Kim in Mississippi also was mistreated at the abortion clinic:

After taking a sedative and being strapped to the exam table I said, "I can't do this. Let me up." After that, I was forcefully held down by two people and given another sedative, this time an injection in the vein in my hand. I put my legs together and heard the doctor tell his assistant to do something about that. They held my legs apart and I begged and called for my boyfriend. Today, I know that he never heard my screams. The doctor started the procedure and I felt pain and could hear the suction noise. I felt sick and could feel the hot tears flowing down my face. I just wanted to die.

In Kentucky, Vicki fared no better.

At the abortion clinic, we were given no counseling. They gave us a standard medical form to fill out and that was it. No one discussed with us that we had other options. No one spoke to us about adoption or parenting.

They just asked about our money. When the procedure began, I asked the doctor to stop and he said to me "Shut up little girl. You should have thought of that before you got yourself knocked up." I have never been treated so poorly in my entire life.

These are just a fraction of the testimonies on the Silent No More Awareness Campaign website and I encourage you to read more. They are first-hand accounts of the pain and suffering caused by abortion.

Equally powerful are the testimonies of those who worked inside abortion clinics and have since left. Nancy Zevgolis is a nurse who exercised her rights of conscience to avoid taking part in abortion. She told me her story. One day at a New York City hospital, she was forced to participate in a late-term abortion. Years later, she said, the image is seared into her memory: the doctor, his foot on the operating room table to get better leverage, tearing a full-term baby apart piece by piece with his forceps.

"It comes back to haunt me," said Ms. Zevgolis. "I can still see the baby's rib cage, and the doctor with his foot on the bottom of the table, pulling out parts."

Ms. Zevgolis, a nurse for twenty-seven years at the time, was asked just to prepare the operating room. A young Orthodox Jewish couple, told their baby's heart problems would prove fatal, made the decision to abort at eight-and-a-half months.

"You could see it was hard on them and I remember thinking 'just have the baby and see what happens, you never know.'" Ms. Zevgolis said, "Sometimes I just sit and cry about it."

Although she had said she would not scrub for the procedure, when her replacement didn't arrive and the patient was under anesthesia, she said, "I couldn't leave. I let it go too far."

The bloody abortion took about twenty minutes, and when it was over both she and the other nurse in the room were crying. The parents had to have the baby's parts for a Jewish burial, and Ms. Zevgolis found herself guarding the remains and "hand-carrying them up to pathology." She never knew if the baby was a boy or a girl.

She got dressed and left after that, never returning to that hospital again. But the memories will never leave her. Almost a decade later, she still struggles to comprehend the brutality she witnessed.

"I went to confession because I took part in that," said the devout Catholic. "But even now I still don't feel clean. It just really bothers me in my heart and soul."

Patricia Sandoval from Southern California talked to me about her experience as a clinic worker in one of the many Planned Parenthood facilities in the Los Angeles area.

After having three abortions herself, Ms. Sandoval went to work for Planned Parenthood. The organization was looking for a bilingual employee, and being fluent in English and Spanish, she was hired right away. She was told the facility performed about forty abortions every week, twenty on Wednesday and twenty on Friday.

Her minimal training consisted of a very stern admonishment to "never call it a 'baby.' Never call it a 'he' or a 'she.' Call it an 'it' or a sac of tissue." She was also encouraged to do everything in her power to ensure that every woman came back on abortion day. She was instructed to tell the women that she had had an abortion herself, and that she had come out OK.

Ms. Sandoval's first job was to counsel women during their initial appointments. But on the first abortion day, she was told to accompany the women during the procedures. Her instructions were clear: "Never tell a woman that we throw her baby away in the garbage."

The first patient she accompanied was about three and a half months pregnant. After the procedure, it was her job to take the bag containing the baby, tissue, and blood into a back room, dump out the contents onto a huge Petri dish, and search for body parts. When she could identify all the body parts, Sandoval—a brand new employee with minimal training—then declared the abortion complete.

While examining the parts, she could clearly see the baby's knuckles, the hair on its legs, and the baby's eyebrows and eye lashes. "I could see the baby," she said. She didn't last long at Planned Parenthood; the emotional trauma was too much to bear.

Patricia's experience is not an isolated case. If you would like to read more about people who worked

in the abortion industry, go to www.prolifeaction.org
/providers.

In the summer of 2015, a series of undercover videos
surfaced that suggested that Planned Parenthood was
illegally selling the organs and limbs of aborted babies.
The Center for Medical Progress was responsible for
this sting. You can visit www.babybodyparts.com to view
these videos and the latest on the investigation that was
launched.

Planned Parenthood claimed that the women
donated their baby's body parts willingly but that is not
the case. That is contrary to what the women of the
Silent No More Campaign can attest to. Here's just one
of their stories from Nancy Tanner of the Campaign.

> I already had two little girls and had just started dat-
> ing the man who would become my second husband.
> When I told him I was pregnant, I was expecting him
> to say we would make it work. But he said it was my
> choice and he would pay for the abortion.
>
> I saw my regular doctor at Kaiser and he referred
> me to Planned Parenthood. Kaiser even made the
> appointment for me and arranged for my insurance
> to cover it.
>
> I was a teacher and I had the day off for a Jew-
> ish Holiday the day I went to a Planned Parenthood
> in Washington, D.C. That abortuary is not open
> anymore.
>
> Outside, there was a pro-life woman who handed
> me a rose. That was the only love I saw all day. But
> the first thing they did at Planned Parenthood was

take my rose away. They said they would hold it for me.

As I was filling out paperwork, I saw a permission slip that dealt with disposal of the "products of conception." It said Planned Parenthood could dispose the tissue as they wished. I said I didn't want to sign it, and they said I had to or I couldn't have the abortion. I didn't want my baby to be used for scientific research and I was told "don't worry, it's not a baby." I told her I had two daughters already and I knew what a baby was. What she said next was very revealing, but I didn't realize it at that time. She said, "We don't think it's a baby."

I had changed my mind and I was looking for a way out of going through with the abortion, so I thought about not signing the consent form. But the Planned Parenthood staffer told me that "what you think of as a baby will be used for something good." She asked me if I was an organ donor and I replied I was. She said this was a similar value and that I should give honor to what I thought was my child by signing it. I signed the form.

The room where they killed my child was cold and dirty. I was on the table but wanted to leave and I was pushed back down and they said that it was too late to change my mind. They said it would be quick and painless and I would be fine.

When the doctor came in, he said nothing to me, he just jammed this thing inside me saying "you will feel a little pressure." I heard the horrible sound of the machine that would suck my baby from my womb.

I can still hear it. I hear it now. The cramping was horrific. I felt as if my insides were being torn out. I cried and the nurse said I should take her hand and squeeze it. She pushed me down on the table when I tried to sit up.

Right next to me, at eye level, was a jar connected to the vacuum and I saw it fill up with fluid and blood. This was my baby. I wanted to die.

After that machine was finally turned off, the doctor took the jar and right in front of me, he dumped the contents onto a tray and started looking for the pieces of my baby. "I can't find all the parts," he said, "how pregnant were you?" He yelled at me! "If you get an infection it's not my fault." Then he turned the machine on and vacuumed some more. That was worse than the first time.

The doctor left and told a woman to look for the parts. I was crying and wanted to use my tears to baptize my baby. The woman told me not to worry. "I baptize all the babies," she said. It gave me comfort to think that she would do that, but I thought how bizarre that someone involved in the death of my child would care about his or her soul.

In the recovery room, we were laid out on canvas cots. Most of the women were crying and wouldn't look at each other but the one next to me told me she had just had her sixth abortion. She said she never intended to get pregnant, but whenever she did, she would just make an appointment. She advised me that when I left, I should bury the memory deep and

it would never bother me, until the next time I had an
abortion. I knew then I would never be back.

When I left, I stopped at the desk and asked
for my tissue donation consent form back because I
wanted to rip it up. They told me "it's too late, we
don't have it anymore." I asked for my rose back
and was told they had thrown it away because it was
upsetting the other women. They gave me a phone
number to call if I ran a high fever.

The pro-lifer with the roses was gone when I left.

My abortion wasn't quick, and it wasn't painless, and I wasn't fine. I'm still not fine. I have been
through healing, and I am very active in pro-life now,
but it has been very hard to watch the Planned Parenthood videos. I want to look away, but I won't let
myself. I see that baby whose remains were poured
into a dish, and I remember that's what my baby
looked like.

To know that Planned Parenthood is still doing
this and selling baby body parts and still getting away
with it makes me so angry. It's not for good, it's for
money. I think of all of us in Silent No More; we have
all been through healing and yet this is devastating
for us. What must it be doing to women who haven't
been to healing programs? I can't imagine how much
this must hurt no matter how deeply they have buried
their abortion experiences. It's an indelible memory
that hurts us all. It doesn't go away.

The testimonies of these post-abortive women and
former abortion workers are vital to the pro-life effort.

Like many physicians I know, I didn't want to do them, but it was still legal and it was a woman's right, and I encountered many patients in my practice who had unplanned pregnancies and who requested them. I also began to notice that about third of my patients had had abortions and many of them expressed regret about having had them.

I discovered an interesting thing, too, at that time because I would ask them for the year of their abortion, and I discovered that when they gave me the date that many of them did not give me merely the year, they gave me the exact date of their abortions as easily as most women recall the birthdates of their babies.

Eventually Dr. Hill's conscience won the battle and he stopped doing abortions completely

Dr. Tony Levatino was in practice with several other obstetrician/gynecologists in upstate New York:

During my residency, at least once, sometimes twice a week, I would be the resident whose turn it was to sit down and do the four, five, or six suction D & C [Dilation and Cutterage] abortions that morning. When the abortionist finishes a suction D & C, he has to open a little suction bag and he has to literally reassemble the child. He has to do that because he wants to make sure he didn't leave anything behind.

I had complications, just like everybody else. I have had perforated uteruses. I have had all kinds of problems—bleeding, infection—Lord knows how many of those women are sterile now.

Dr. Levatino admits to having aborted thousands of babies during those years prior to his conversion to the pro-life cause.

Often, pro-lifers focus on the killing of unborn children, and rightfully so. It should not be overlooked, however, that every abortion has two primary victims: the baby and the mother who made her "choice." More than 50 million unborn children have been killed since *Roe v. Wade* and *Doe v. Bolton* legalized abortion-on-demand through all nine months of pregnancy. We will never know how many millions of mothers have suffered, and are suffering still, from the physical and emotional wounds of their abortions. We will never know the full physical, emotional, or psychological consequences of abortion, or how many have died from the after-effects of a botched abortion. But we do know this: abortion is a bad product, and it needs to be recalled.

In 1906, President Theodore Roosevelt signed the Pure Food and Drug Act to protect Americans from the bogus and dangerous products being peddled by unscrupulous entrepreneurs. In 1938, Congress passed the Food, Drug and Cosmetic Act to give teeth to consumer regulations. In 1972, Congress created the Consumer Product Safety Commission, which began its oversight of consumer products the following year—the same year abortion became legal. Tens of thousands of medications and products have been recalled since then, all because they were deemed unsafe—even deadly—for consumers.

The recall of products extends well beyond health care, of course. And recalls are routinely instituted for products that cause far, far fewer deaths and injuries than in a pool of her own blood, her pulse racing and her blood pressure dangerously low. The woman, identified only as Angela P. in records of the Medical Board of California, had gone to the Clinica Medica Para la Mujer de Hoy in Santa Ana in the summer of 2004 for an abortion.

Dr. Phillip Rand, then in his early 80s, performed a vaginal suction procedure, despite having determined that Angela was about 20 weeks pregnant, well into her second trimester. She was given no anesthesia or painkillers. Angela P.'s experience was cited in a 2004 medical board accusation against Rand as "barbaric" and a "severe departure" from a reasonable standard of care. Rand surrendered his license in 2005.

Rand was one of at least six doctors with histories of malpractice complaints, addiction or medical board actions who were employed by a chain of Southern California abortion clinics, according to court and medical board records. Now Bertha Bugarin, 48, who authorities say manages the clinics, has been charged with practicing medicine without a license on five patients in February and March 2007, according to a statement from Los Angeles County District Attorney, Steve Cooley's office.[5]

In 2006 in Florida, there was a similar case. According to a Health Grades background check on the abortionist:

The patient, while waiting for the physician to arrive at the clinic, delivered a live fetus and one of the owners of the clinic placed the fetus and all of its remains in a closed plastic bag and placed it in a trashcan. The police obtained a search warrant of the clinic and found the partially decomposed fetal remains in a cardboard box. The physician failed to secure the services of another physician to care for the patient while the patient was in active labor while the physician was not present at the clinic and failed to arrange for 911 to transfer the patient to a hospital. The physician also failed to ensure the proper disposal of the fetus.

The physician, Dr. Pierre Renelique also failed to keep adequate medical records justifying the patient's course of treatment. This physician falsified the patient's medical records by indicating that a dilation and extraction abortion was performed when the patient had already delivered the fetus. He also delegated professional responsibilities to an individual who was not qualified or licensed to perform. The physician ordered unlicensed personnel to start an IV to administer medications.[6]

In another case, the Metropolitan Medical Associates in Englewood, New Jersey, one of the state's largest abortion clinics, reached a $1.9 million settlement with a woman who suffered massive hemorrhaging, a coma, and a stroke after she had an abortion at the facility in 2007. She would later require a hysterectomy. After the incident was reported, state inspectors found dirty forceps, rusty crochet hooks used to remove IUDs, and a quarter-inch of dark red "dirt and debris" under an examining table in the Engle Street clinic. The state allowed the facility to reopen in March 2007.[7]

Abortion doctors who engage in unsafe and unsanitary practices do often have their licenses revoked. The problem, however, is that just as often they simply move on to another state. All the while, women remain at serious risk.

"Women are in far more danger today than they have ever been," says Troy Newman, president of Operation Rescue, a Wichita, Kansas, organization that investigates abortion malpractice. "The level of incompetence among abortionists is higher than ever and the complication rate is extraordinary."

It's clear that despite being legal, abortion is neither rare, nor safe for women.

Because the abortion industry, often in collusion with government agencies, is so skilled at covering its tracks we may never know for sure how many women have been injured or killed after choosing abortion. One thing is clear: the more we dig, the more we find.

*   *   *   *   *

Abortion supporters often dismiss claims that abortion harms women, but those who have been through the nightmare of abortion tell stories that no one can refute. Kelly Clinger is one of these women.

Ms. Clinger is a singer, recording artist, and spokeswoman for the Silent No More Awareness Campaign. In 2000, she had an abortion at fifteen weeks at a clinic run by Dr. James Pendergaft in Orlando.

Clinger recalls her abortion:

It was like a cattle call. It was dirty. I couldn't take anything with me, not even a purse. The only thing I could bring was a cell phone and cash, because you have to pay in cash there. We were hustled in, one after another. I was put under for the abortion and when I woke up I was in a recliner in a room with about 25 other girls. Everyone was crying, and they were trying to give us crackers and juice. They gave me some instructions about what to look for, and I went home.

Two or three weeks after the abortion, I had very heavy bleeding. I had had an abortion before, so I knew this was unusual. I made an appointment with my ob/gyn and I decided not to tell her I had just had an abortion. She did some tests, and then told me I had to have a cone biopsy, which tests for cervical cancer.

It was about four weeks after the abortion. I was put under general anesthesia. When I woke up, my doctor was standing next to the table I was lying on, and she was crying. She told me she knew I had an abortion because she found parts of the baby still inside me. She had to do a D&C (dilation and curettage) to get the parts of the baby out. She also discovered that the doctor had torn my uterus apart. She wasn't sure I would ever be able to carry a baby to term. After I got married, I did get pregnant and I gave birth, but they told me—and now I don't know if it was even true—that it would be detrimental to my life to bear more children. I had my tubes tied.

Pendergaft has served time in Federal prison for extortion and perjury and his medical license has been suspended four times in Florida. In 2011, he was ordered to pay $36.7 million to a former patient at his clinic for malpractice. In 2015, Pendergraft was arrested in South Carolina during a traffic stop where police found drugs and forceps covered in blood and human tissue. This led police to believe that he was operating an illegal mobile abortion business. As of this writing, his clinic in Orlando is still in operation and still performs late-term abortions.

*   *   *   *   *

Deborah Cardamone knows all too well the complications of abortion. She lost her only child, Marla, to a legal abortion performed in a well-known, highly regarded women's hospital in Pittsburgh.

After giving birth to a baby boy at fifteen, Marla was the victim of date rape at eighteen and got pregnant again. At the time, she was being treated for bipolar disorder. Her mother was helping to raise Marla's son, Julian, and caring for Marla's quadriplegic father. A social worker told Marla it would be unfair to expect her mother to help with the new baby on top of everything else. But Deborah and her husband begged their daughter to have the baby and said they would help raise him or help make an adoption plan, if that's what Marla wanted.

"She was able to put the social worker off for a couple of weeks," Deborah recalled, "but when they got her in for another appointment, she was told the medication she was taking for her depression would cause heart and brain damage to the baby. They said the baby would not have a chance. Everything seemed so bleak to her and she was so fragile."

When she was seventeen weeks pregnant, Marla met with a doctor she had never seen before for an abortion that began with an injection of urea into her womb and the insertion of laminaria to dilate her cervix. She was put on an intravenous drip of Pitocin to induce labor.

"When that was over, I walked with her to her room," Deborah said. "She crawled into bed and said, 'that really hurt.'"

Deborah stayed with her until 11 p.m. She remembers thinking how tiny Marla looked in the bed. It was the last time she would see her alive.

The next morning, Deborah got a call from a nurse in the intensive care unit, telling her something had gone wrong and that both she and her husband should rush to the hospital. They were not able to arrange transportation for Marla's father so Deborah went alone.

"When I got to Marla's room, a nurse turned me around and pushed me out of the room," Deborah said. "I begged to see her. When they asked me if I had other children, I lost all my breath, all my hope. I was within ten feet of my only child but they wouldn't let me see her. They denied me everything because a cover-up had to start."

Deborah finally was allowed to see Marla just prior to an autopsy.

"I could not tell it was my daughter, except for her hair," she recalled. "Her face was swollen and purple.

Her eyes were yellow. She was 30 pounds heavier. It was the most horrific thing I had ever seen, and I see that in my head every day."

Following their successful lawsuit against the doctors and the hospital, the grieving parents learned the horrific circumstances of Marla's death. The official cause of death was sepsis from an induced abortion, but the massive infection claimed her life before she had delivered her stillborn son. The baby was removed during the autopsy, and Marla's parents naturally assumed he was replaced in her womb before Marla was buried. But Marla was buried alone; her son was disposed of as medical waste.

"This was not a back alley abortion," Deborah said. "This was a big hospital with a big reputation."

Whenever Deborah hears abortion described as vital health care for women, she said, "I see a picture of my daughter after her death. When I hear women buying that lie, I hurt for them."

*   *   *   *   *

Laura Hope Smith was twenty-two-years-old and engaged to be married to a soldier serving in Iraq when she decided to have an abortion. Accompanied by a friend, she went to an abortion clinic in Hyannis, Massachusetts, owned by Rapin Osathanondh, a one-time Harvard fellow who by then was using his medical training solely to perform abortions and to teach other abortionists his techniques.

Osathanondh administered Propofol to Laura (the

same powerful anesthetic that killed Michael Jackson), performed the abortion, and then left her in the care of his only office worker, a woman with no medical training. Laura never regained consciousness. Not realizing his patient had died during the abortion, Osathanondh went on to perform the procedure on his next victim.

"Laura died during the murder of my grandchild and he didn't even notice," says Laura's mother, Eileen Smith. "When you're in the killing business, you don't pay much attention to life."

By law, Propofol must be administered in a hospital and only by an anesthesiologist. After the office worker called 911 for Laura, emergency medical technicians had to move her to a hallway to try to revive her, because the abortion room was no bigger than a closet.

The Smiths pursued criminal and civil charges against the abortionist, and on the third anniversary of Laura's death, he went to jail to serve a three-month sentence.

"Michael Vick got two years for killing dogs," Mrs. Smith said, referring to the much-publicized case of an NFL quarterback who was involved with dog-fighting. "The man who murdered my daughter got three months."

Unlike all the publicity surrounding Vick's arrest, after Laura was killed during an abortion, it took her local paper, the *Cape Cod Times*, six weeks to run a story.

Mrs. Smith and her husband had adopted Laura after the girl was abandoned in an orphanage in her native Honduras and then abused by her first adoptive parents. The Smiths got a phone call about a little girl who needed help. Twenty-two years later, they received a call telling them that little girl was gone.

"Laura came into my life with a phone call, and she left with a phone call," says her mother, whose heartache will never heal.

Tragically, the abortion clinic where Laura was killed was next door to a pro-life pregnancy medical clinic where she could have seen a sonogram of her unborn baby and found help and hope, instead of death. The clinic is part a group of Boston area centers called A Woman's Concern, affiliated with Heartbeat International. It opened next door to the abortion clinic so that girls like Laura would not have only one option. As Dr. Peggy Hartshorn, President of Heartbeat International, said:

> I have consulted with so many girls like Laura who are from strong Christian families, yet they think their only option is abortion because of their fear and shame about disappointing their parents or church community. As parents, we need to tell our kids over and over, "Nothing you can say or do will make me stop loving you." Churches need to give the same message, "Nothing you can do can make Jesus stop loving you."

Laura's story did not end with her death from abortion, God brought good out of it. Our clinic on the Cape, A Woman's Concern, was having its annual banquet only four days after her tragic death, and the staff reached out to her parents. Mrs. Smith came to the banquet and was welcomed and ministered to. The clinic kept in close contact with the family, offering support and healing, as we do with anyone who has been touched by abortion. Mrs. Smith, within a year, came to our Heartbeat International conference and met with many people in our movement. She has done great good by sharing her daughter's story at events, schools, and colleges. She has become a powerful witness on the dangers of so-called "safe, legal" abortion.

Now you might be saying to yourself, "Oh these are isolated cases that happened years ago. The abortion industry must have cleaned up its act by now, right?" Wrong! Abortion is not getting any safer for women.

In July 2012, a twenty-four-year-old Chicago woman died following a second trimester abortion at a Planned Parenthood clinic in Chicago.

The *Chicago Tribune* reported that Tonya Reaves died on July 20 after she began to bleed heavily, according to the Cook County medical examiner's office. Her death was ruled an accident.

The victim's twin sister told a Chicago radio station that her family wants answers.

"It happened so fast," said Toni Reaves. "She was just fine one day—and then the next day she was gone. We're just trying to figure out what happened."

Dorsey Johns, Tonya's mother, filed a wrongful death lawsuit against Planned Parenthood in August of 2012. The suit alleges that Planned Parenthood failed to call 911 immediately and allowed Tonya to bleed profusely for more than five hours before taking her to the emergency room. Doctors at the hospital had to perform a second abortion when they discovered the first one was incomplete.

This is just a snapshot of the horrors taking place

to find baby parts inside a woman following an abortion. They had seen it all before.

Next time you hear the antiseptic term "incomplete abortion," think of this young woman and what was done to her in an abortion clinic. No, abortion is not safe or rare, but it is legal.

Isn't it time to recall abortion?

CHAPTER FOUR

CHILDREN MADE TO ORDER

CONSIDER WHAT the architects of legalized abortion promised it would do for women and for society as a whole. They said that there would be no more unwanted children. Women would be in control of their reproductive lives and they could have their careers. They could delay marriage and childbirth until they were truly ready. The stated (and misleading) goal was to make every child a wanted child, born at a time when the parents felt they were ready both financially and emotionally to start their family.

Almost thirty years after abortion became legal, the Alan Guttmacher Institute (the research arm of Planned Parenthood) was still spouting this optimism about how abortion had improved the lives of children. Here's an excerpt from a 2002 Guttmacher report. "Abortion legalization may have led to an improvement in the average living conditions of children, probably by reducing the numbers of youngsters who would have lived in single-parent families, lived in poverty, received welfare and died as infants."[1]

Probably? Probably not.

Here is the 2010 report from the Children's Defense Fund, a non-profit child advocacy organization:

> Whether looking at poverty, health coverage, family structure, family income, early childhood development, education, child abuse and neglect, juvenile justice, or gun violence, the news is mostly not good for the children, their families, or the fabric of the future of our nation. Millions of children continue in or to be at risk of entering the cradle-to-prison pipeline. This crisis threatens the well-being and future of poor children of color across our nation.[2]

The report shows that there were 11.5 million children living in poverty in 1980, and 14.1 million in 2010. Legal abortion clearly did not solve the problem of poverty, but it did change the way we look at children.

Contraception is sold to women as a tool for them to control their reproductive health. And when their contraception fails, abortion allows them to get rid of their unwanted and unplanned pregnancy. This contraceptive mentality leaves children in a precarious situation. If they are "wanted," they are seen as a blessing, a miracle, a tiny bundle of unlimited potential. If they are unwanted, they are nothing but a parasite, a "product of conception" that can be emptied from the unwilling mother's uterus. In reality, of course, a baby is a baby, wanted or otherwise. But pro-aborts have been conditioned to believe that their desire, their choice, is what determines a child's humanity. Hence, the oft-proclaimed mantra: "My body, my choice."

For decades after *Roe v. Wade*, the pro-choice

movement held fast to its assertion that a baby in the womb is just a blob of tissue or cells. But the advent of ultrasound technology made it impossible to continue selling that lie to women. In fact, in pregnancy help medical clinics today, where women who are considering abortion can see their unborn baby via ultrasound, many women choose life! Almost everyone has seen an ultrasound picture of a baby in the womb. No doubt, the "contents of the uterus" is an unborn baby. Now, the argument of the pro-choice camp becomes, "the rights of the mother trump those of her unborn child."

That a unique human life begins at conception is a scientific fact, not a religious argument. It follows that a child's human rights also begin at conception, but pro-abortion groups continue to dismiss the rights of unborn children. So much for improving the "living" conditions of children.

*   *   *   *   *

Having turned conception and childbirth into something to be wholly manipulated at will, more and more women are delaying marriage and childbirth in favor of higher education and career advancement. But this delay is causing them to sacrifice their most fertile years.

The median age for a woman's first marriage was 26.1 years in 2010, up from 23.9 in 1990, and up from 22.0 in 1980.[3]

Once married, many women delay starting their families well into their 30s, and then they routinely encounter difficulties becoming pregnant. Couples often find themselves turning to reproductive technologies like in vitro fertilization (IVF), a radical and unnatural procedure that only those going through it—and those profiting from it—truly understand.

Let me pause briefly to address the morality of IVF in itself before we get to some of the truly horrific practical outcomes. The Catholic Church teaches that any kind of reproductive technology that separates conception from the sexual union of wives and husbands is wrong. Two documents—*Instruction on Respect for Human Life* and *Dignitatis Personae*—eloquently explain the Church's position, and I urge you to read them for yourself. Both can be found on the Vatican website.[4]

Put simply and briefly, the Church teaches that when we separate conception from the act of marital love—as IVF certainly does—then we begin to go off course, as individuals and as a society. When we use IVF, we are treating our own bodies like incubators and our children like commodities. That attitude toward children, toward life itself, explains what can come next in the life of an IVF baby.

Here are the basics of how IVF works: A man's sperm and a woman's egg are combined in a laboratory dish, where fertilization occurs. The resulting embryo is then transferred to the woman's uterus to implant and develop naturally. Usually, two to four embryos are placed in the uterus to increase the chances of a successful implantation.

About 63 percent of IVF pregnancies result in single babies, 32 percent result in twins, and 5 percent result in triplets or more. It is no longer rare for IVF women to have quadruplets or quintuplets. Who hasn't heard of "Octomom"?

The IVF procedure often is not covered by insurance companies, and it can cost $10,000 or more per cycle. Clearly, IVF "produces" wanted children. But it also produces unwanted children.

Extraordinary means were used to achieve conception, but what if a procedure was *too* successful? What if there are more children than a couple wants?

Selective reduction is the next step in this reproductive odyssey. Imagine a couple that has desperately tried to conceive a child, and has devoted months, even years, of their time in addition to tens of thousands of dollars to having a baby. Now, suppose they discover that the mother is carrying two or more babies in her womb. Couples are often counseled that they can have the family they want simply by agreeing to kill one or more of the children they worked so hard to conceive. It's called "selective reduction" and it is usually done twelve to fourteen weeks into the pregnancy.

You might be wondering how a couple chooses which baby to "reduce." If the woman is pregnant with twins and both babies are healthy, the doctor usually terminates the baby who is easiest to reach with a needle of potassium chloride, which causes the baby's heart to stop. If the babies are different sexes, then the doctor may ask the couple which child they want to keep, the boy or the girl. It is an everyday occurrence in very reputable hospitals around the country.

In an August 2011 *New York Times Magazine* article, "The Two Minus One Pregnancy," a woman who

reduced her twins to a singleton summed up with horrific clarity where contraception, abortion, and reproductive technologies have led us as a society. This is what
"Jenny" told journalist Ruth Padawer:

> If I had conceived these twins naturally, I wouldn't
> have reduced this pregnancy, because you feel like if
> there's a natural order, then you don't want to disturb
> it. But we created this child in such an artificial man-
> ner—in a test tube, choosing an egg donor, having
> the embryo placed in me—and somehow, making a
> decision about how many to carry seemed to be just
> another choice. The pregnancy was all so consumer-
> ish to begin with, and this became yet another thing
> we could control.[5]

Ms. Padawer's eye-opening article also followed a
physician who specialized in IVF. As Dr. Robert Evans
began doing reductions of large numbers of babies down
to twins, he saw the need for the development of ethical guidelines. But by 2004, with improvements in ultrasound technology and IVF successes for older women,
he began to advocate for the reduction of twins to sin-
gletons. "Ethics," he was quoted in the *Times Magazine*
article, "evolve with technology."

When I read the article I was outraged, initially on the
basis of the moral issues but also because I was a mother of
twins. I had one daughter who was twenty-three-months
old when I gave birth to twin girls. Sonograms were a
new technology back in the early 1980s so I wasn't aware
that I was carrying twins until the final month of pregnancy. I clearly remember the panic: How would I take

care of twins and my twenty-three-month-old daughter? I understand what these mothers are feeling.

But instead of turning to doctors who are all too ready to kill the unwanted brother or sister of the wanted baby, what these women really need is to surround themselves with people who will help them handle this new adventure. In fact, there are support groups for mothers of multiples. I was involved with a group like this and I am greatly appreciative of their "been there, done that, and survived" attitude!

The pro-choice crowd will often retort that pro-lifers are hypocritical in condemning IVF. Shouldn't all women be able to have children? Shouldn't we encourage new life? Well, there are other ways to promote fertility, naturally and morally, that don't involve treating women's bodies as farms, and treating babies like a litter, where one is picked and the rest are discarded.

When pro-lifers warn couples off the path of IVF and selective reduction, it is not to quash their hope that they will ever have a family. There is a solution that is both morally acceptable and better for the heath of women. It is called NaPro Technology, a healthy and practical way of approaching a woman's problems with infertility.

I had an opportunity to interview NaPro Technology practitioner Dr. Anne Nolte of the Gianna Center for Women's Health and Fertility in Manhattan, where women's menstrual problems and fertility struggles are treated as medical problems, as they should be.

When I had heavy periods as a teenager, my doctor put me on the Pill. That's the easy way out for doctors, according to Dr. Nolte:

When the Pill came along, doctors no longer needed
to look for the "why." Why do some women have very
heavy periods? Why are some women so irregular?
The answer now is just to shut down the system with
the Pill, rather than to find out what's going wrong
and treat that. We don't do that in any other area of
medicine. It is shockingly bad medicine. The Catholic Church gets a bad rap on contraception but in fact,
from a medical perspective, good ethics have actually
led to better medicine.

Irregularities in the menstrual cycle mean something
might be wrong, that something is not working the way
it's supposed to. Physicians like Dr. Nolte, who practice
their faith on the job, look for the cause of the problem
and work to treat it, either with medicines or hormonal
therapies. IVF, on the other hand, skips the diagnosis,
ignores the potential medical problems with women,
and often "creates" unwanted children who are summar-
ily eliminated.

Advances in the area of natural family planning
ultimately led to the development of NaPro Technology. "Doctors and scientists trying to be faithful to the
Church discovered that the natural family planning chart
could also be a diagnostic tool for infertility," Dr. Nolte
said. "Like irregular periods, infertility is a symptom
of something—hormonal problems, anatomical problems—that are often correctable."

Dr. Nolte said 95 percent of the couples who come to
her with difficulty conceiving or who are suffering recur-
rent miscarriage have no diagnosis when they arrive, and

a majority of them have their problems diagnosed and treated and are able to conceive and carry to term.

"Our success rate is as good or better than IVF," she said. "And we have very low rates of multiple births, and very low rates of birth defects."

The one area where NaPro Technology pales in comparison to IVF is that no one is getting rich off it. "We actually lose money," Dr. Nolte said.

When considering IVF, couples should be aware that there are better alternatives for women that are both beneficial to their health and morally acceptable.*

For many of us, selective reduction is too horrible to contemplate. But the harsh reality is that often the creation of a "wanted" child comes at the expense of creating and killing an unwanted child. And it's a reality that an increasing number of couples are choosing. What are the consequences for parents who choose IVF and selective reduction? What kind of lasting affect will it have on the surviving baby?

Parents may suffer crippling guilt, knowing that they deliberately chose to terminate the life of one of their children while keeping the other child. Imagine every birthday and special occasion, looking at the chosen child and remembering the child or children who were killed in that same shared womb.

Parents can attempt to shut off their emotions and to ignore their conscience but the reality and the consequences will not go away. Consider, for example, this

---

* To find a medical consultant like Dr. Nolte, go to www.fertility care.org

quote from the *New York Times Magazine* article on selective reduction:

> A New York woman was certain that she wanted to reduce from twins to a singleton. Her husband yielded because she would be the one carrying the pregnancy and would stay at home to raise them. They came up with a compromise. "I asked not to see any of the ultrasounds," he said. "I didn't want to have that image, the image of two. I didn't want to torture myself. And I didn't go in for the procedure either, because less is more for me." His wife was relieved that her husband remained in the waiting room; she, too, didn't want to deal with his feelings.

The problem is that these couples, like it or not, will have to deal with their feelings, eventually. At some point, they will have to confront their conscience.

Kevin Burke, cofounder of Rachel's Vineyard, has noted:

> Couples who end up playing God with the lives of their unborn children not only violate the moral law; they also violate something fundamental to their identity as parents; the protection of their offspring. I have discovered in our work with healing after abortions that men, in particular, suffer very profound grief, depression and anxiety when they participate in reduction decisions and procedures. They may try and distance themselves from the horror to escape the consequences of silencing the natural desire to protect their unborn child.

These fathers experience a very traumatic death experience that will leave them and their marriages deeply wounded as they acknowledge their actions were wrong and they deeply regret their decision.

Now consider for a moment the surviving child. Many studies have been conducted about the lives of twins in utero. Recently, Italian researchers found that by fourteen weeks twins begin making movements directed at their sibling. The babies were seen intentionally touching their twin's eye and mouth regions and were even seen "caressing" the back of their sibling. By the eighteenth week, the researchers calculated that 30 percent of all the babies' movements were directed specifically at their twin, and those movements were more accurate and longer in duration than self-directed movements.[6] Now keep in mind that most selective reductions occur from the fourteenth week and even later if sex selection is a factor. The surviving baby knows his or her sibling has been lost.

Similarly, there are psychological effects on siblings of aborted children. Dr. Philip Ney, a Canadian psychologist, has studied these effects for decades. He tells a story of a woman who came to him for counseling for her six-year-old child who was having nightmares, wetting the bed, and suffering from separation anxiety. Dr. Ney, in his interview with the mother, asked her about any pregnancy losses. She told him about two abortions that she had prior to giving birth to this child. Then in a separate interview with the child, Dr. Ney asked the child to draw a picture of her family. She was an only child, and yet she drew a picture with her Mom, Dad, a brother, a sister, and herself. She had a sense of the missing siblings.

"What is it like to grow up in a home where you suspect or you know that one of your little unborn siblings was aborted?" Dr. Ney asked. "It creates a whole range of very, very deep conflicts. And we now call that post-abortion survivor syndrome." Dr. Ney continued:

> They (abortion survivors) have in common many of the conflicts that were found in those people who survived the Holocaust. For instance they have survivor guilt. They feel it is not right for them to be alive. And they wonder why they should be selected when their little siblings were selected to die . . . which is precisely what happened to the people from the Holocaust. Why were they selected to live and some of their friends, relatives, and family were selected to die? And it leaves this deep sense of guilt.

Survivor anxiety is another symptom these survivors struggle with. They escaped death once, but now fear it lurking behind every corner, ready to spring out at them. This and the rest of the constellation of symptoms can make it very difficult for survivors to trust, hope, build confident relationships, and plan for their futures.

Not only do abortion, IVF, and selective reduction fail at ensuring that every child is a wanted child, but they also cause damage to mothers, fathers, and surviving siblings.

Isn't it time that we recall abortion?

CHAPTER FIVE

HAVING IT ALL: HAVE WE REALLY COME A LONG WAY, BABY?

TO DETERMINE how far women have traveled along the path to equal rights, we need to take a look back in history. Let's go back to the early American feminists.

One of the first feminists was Susan B. Anthony. Born on February 15, 1820, in Adams, Massachusetts, Anthony was brought up in a Quaker family with deep activist traditions. Early in her life she developed a sense of justice and moral zeal. After teaching for fifteen years, she became active in the temperance movement. But because she was a woman, she was not allowed to speak at temperance rallies.

This experience, and her acquaintance with Elizabeth Cady Stanton, a prominent activist, led her to join the women's rights movement in 1852. Soon after, she dedicated her life to women's suffrage. She traveled the country giving lectures and campaigning for the right for women to vote. She also fought for the abolition of slavery and the right for women to own property and retain their earnings.

Susan B. Anthony was also pro-life. Even though she never married or had children, she viewed children as a blessing. In a letter to fellow suffragist, Frances Willard, Anthony wrote, "Sweeter even than to have had the joy of children of my own has it been for me to help bring about a better state of things for mothers generally, so that their unborn little ones could not be willed away from them."[1]

Elizabeth Cady Stanton was also pro-life. In a letter to Julia Ward Howe, the woman who wrote "The Battle Hymn of the Republic," Stanton wrote: "When we consider that women are treated as property, it is degrading to women that we should treat our children as property to be disposed of as we see fit."[2]

These early feminists fought for women's rights but in no way did they consider abortion empowering for women.

Fast forward to the early 1900s. Margaret Sanger, who opened the first birth control clinic in 1916 in New York City, proclaimed that women should be free to have sexual relations as desired and be free from the fear of becoming pregnant. Even Sanger, however, wasn't an advocate for abortion in the early days. In her 1931 essay, "Birth Control Advances: A Reply to the Pope," which she wrote in response to Pope Pius XI's encyclical, *Casti Connubi*, that stressed the sanctity of marriage and prohibited Catholics from using birth control, Sanger stated:

> Although abortion may be resorted to in order to save
> the life of the mother, the practice of it merely for

limitation of offspring is *dangerous and vicious*. I bring up the subject here only because some ill-informed persons have the notion that when we speak of birth control we include abortion as a method. We certainly do not.[3]

In 1952, Planned Parenthood of Iowa distributed a pamphlet on birth control that included a question and answer section on what, exactly, birth control is.

Question: Is it an abortion?

Answer: Definitely not. An abortion requires an operation. *It kills the life of a baby after it has begun.* It is dangerous to your life and health. It may make you sterile so that when you want a child you cannot have it. Birth control merely postpones the beginning of life." [emphasis mine][4]

Of course even this quote is not accurate. The birth control pill doesn't always prevent fertilization. Sometimes it prevents the fertilized embryo from being implanted in the mother's uterus. But the point is that even Margret Sanger and Planned Parenthood once recognized abortion for what it is: murder.

By the 1960s and '70s the atmosphere of the country was changing rapidly: "If you can't be with the one you love, love the one you are with," right? Sex was taken out of the marital act and became recreational. Teenage pregnancies were increasing and therefore Planned Parenthood became society's problem solver.

The U.S. government became partners with Planned Parenthood in 1970, when President Richard Nixon signed the "Title X" bill, which gave government money to the organization for family planning (birth control). The organization still receives our tax dollars, to the tune of about $1 million a day.

So what does Planned Parenthood—which grew out of the feminist movement, and now plays a massive role in society—do for those girls and women who get pregnant even though they are using birth control? It sells them an abortion, which quietly became not only acceptable to the organization, but necessary.

In 1970, Planned Parenthood Syracuse became the first affiliate to add abortion to its services. After 1973 and the passing of *Roe v. Wade* and *Doe v. Bolton*, abortion swept across the country like wildfire. Free-standing abortion clinics began to sprout up in cities all across America, and Planned Parenthood became the number one provider.

The grand irony is that these clinics, born from the feminist movement and operating under the premise of providing women's health, largely serve only to harm women. A woman gets pregnant and feels that she needs to have an abortion. She'll arrive at the clinic either on her own or accompanied by a friend, family member, or maybe the baby's father. But she will go through the procedure all by herself. Furthermore, many abortions are coerced. The baby's father may have told the woman to end the pregnancy or he will end the relationship. Sometimes, perhaps more often than we can ever know, there is a threat of violence. How might that make a woman feel? Planned Parenthood doesn't care. How's that for empowering women and providing for women's health?

Let's hear from some more women who have been down this road.

Milagros, who lives in a U.S. territory, recalls her abortion this way:

> I had an abortion because my boyfriend asked me to. He said he could not have a new baby (he has two). He said that he would not take away his time with his kids to have time with mine. I felt so lost. We had been together for three years. I waited to have the abortion because I wanted to have the baby. I know how it feels to be a mom and it is wonderful. But he started being mean and manipulative, taking my life experiences and his and turning them against me and our future. I felt so lonely, so ashamed. What was supposed to be loved and wanted—a baby—felt so wrong for his future.
>
> He sold a gold chain to pay for the abortion procedure and took me there. The first time I did not go in and went home. It felt so right. He called and said that if I had the baby he could not love it. He made me feel as if the baby and I were going to be in danger. I took a long walk, cried, and asked myself: Will I ever be safe again? What if my baby is abused because he does not want it? Will the law be on my side?

Milagros went through with the abortion.

Melissa from Pennsylvania knew she was pregnant when she couldn't stand the taste of toothpaste at her dentist's office. When she confirmed her suspicions with a pregnancy test, her life took a turn for the worse.

My husband's immediate reaction was, "We discussed this before. We can't afford another." I felt like it was him or the baby. I felt totally helpless. Our marriage was already in trouble. I was the only bread winner and we were already living paycheck to paycheck. . . . I cried a little and then made an appointment, as I wanted to get it over with as quickly as possible.

The abortion clinic I went to treated me like a piece of meat. They didn't have enough seats in the building so half of the time I was forced to stand while I waited. When it was finally my turn, they took me to a back room to change. In the waiting room were five other girls, all naked except for a gown and sheet. The waiting room was also the only room that had a bathroom in it, so fully clothed patients and staff kept walking in and out while I sat there naked, cold and shivering because they had no heat except a tiny space heater.

When it was my turn, I walked down the hall and got on the table. The anesthesiologist was the only one who seemed to care that I was upset. He told me not to worry, he would make sure I didn't feel any pain. When I woke up, he promised, it would all be over.

When I finally met the abortionist, he didn't even say hello to me. The nurse just said "this is doctor . . ." whatever his name was. It's kind of embarrassing to meet your doctor for the first time with your legs in the air.

When I woke up they had me transfer to a recliner. I felt nauseated, but the nurse wouldn't give me anything for nausea. I lied about the nausea when it was time to leave because I just wanted to get out of there. I felt like crap; I knew what I did was wrong. All I could think of was that my precious baby was somewhere in a red bag labeled medical waste.

About a week after the abortion, I ended up at the crisis center of my local hospital as I was severely depressed and having suicidal thoughts.

Jacquie Stalnaker's boyfriend drove her to an abortion clinic with a gun on the floor of the car. He told her their baby would die that day, or that both she and the baby would. When she came out of the clinic afterward, he was nowhere to be found and never seen again. She collapsed on the street and came to in a hospital, where she learned that she had lost half the blood in her body. Years later, she would survive recurring stage-four uterine cancer and the removal of a twenty-five-pound tumor.

Ms. Stalnaker, a former Miss West Virginia, had aborted the only child she would ever conceive. She was twenty-two when she had the abortion and forty-four when she was finally able to talk openly about it and the pain it has caused her.

"Half my life," she said, "was spent in trauma."

Planned Parenthood and other abortion clinics certainly peddle an odd form of women's health care.

After an abortion, a woman often bears the guilt and emotional trauma alone. The physical pain is also hers. Where is the man in all this? Frequently his only contribution is to pay for half of the abortion. If their contraception has failed, abortion is their fail-safe option. Our society has lost the concept of personal responsibility. Years ago, if a man got a girl pregnant, they either got married or made an adoption plan. Now, even married women have abortions and 40 percent of children are born to single mothers. I suppose that means we women have our independence, but we have lost our way.

With a better understanding of their fertility and an array of contraceptive choices available, women have gained control of their reproductive lives. They are delaying marriage and childbirth into their thirties and beyond. They have advanced degrees and corner offices. The glass ceiling, while still there, rises higher and higher. So maybe we do have it all?

Numerous polls in the last several years have shown that, for the first time since pollsters started asking the question, men are now happier than women. The surveys also say that despite their many gains, women are still doing almost all of the housework and child-rearing, whether they work outside the home or not.

So now we have women who have their careers, delay marriage until late into their twenties, and give birth to the first "wanted child" a few years later. After giving birth, they return to work and their baby is either with a Nanny or in day care. Let's look at the typical day for a working Mom.

She rises early, gets herself ready for work, and then deals with her baby and other children—dressing and feeding them and then dropping them off at day care or school. She works all day and then either she or her spouse pick up the children, rush home to make dinner or order takeout, and then dive into the nighttime chores: checking homework, giving baths, putting the children to bed. If she is not too exhausted, there are still dishes to wash and laundry to do. Some husbands help out with these chores, but they also put in a full day at work. This daily grind leaves little or no time for husbands and wives to be together. They collapse into bed with exhaustion, only to hear the sound of the alarm in the morning when the schedule begins again. Now that's great birth control!

These women have bought into the "you can have it all" canard. They meet their Prince Charming, buy and furnish their dream houses, park two cars in the garage and plan fabulous vacations. They say to themselves, "Now we have the perfect children and family life." But look at the schedules they keep. Where's the quality time with children and spouses? Even weekends aren't restful—soccer games, dance recitals, and all the other extracurricular activities we feel so compelled to take part in. Even at dinner, the television is on and everyone is texting on their smart phones.

How is this empowering women?

The national Centers for Disease Control has been tracking marriage, divorce, and family structure since 1973 (coincidentally, the same year that *Roe* and *Doe* legalized abortion). Its 2010 National Survey of Family Growth found that about 50 percent of marriages end in divorce, and that those couples who lived together before marriage had the worst track records.[5]

The reasons for such widespread divorce are many and vary from family to family, but the overarching explanation is that the culture has changed. Commitment and family are no longer paramount. It's all about "me." If an individual is unhappy, unfulfilled, or bored, there is no societal pressure to try to work things out for the good of the family. Our sense of entitlement has grown so strong that anything that gets in the way of the plans we've engineered has to go.

That sense of entitlement goes hand-in-hand with the widespread use of contraception and abortion. A child would be too difficult or would interfere with our plans? Easy, just "take care of it." A woman is made—literally—to be a mother. That doesn't mean women can't work or have careers, but contraception and abortion, far from empowering women, actually serve to snatch away from women the very thing that makes them unique and powerful.

The original feminists of Susan B. Anthony's day fought for the right to vote. When the women's movement of the 1960s began, women were fighting for equal pay and a more level footing with men. But that movement and its noble goals were hijacked by those who saw abortion as the great equalizer. Forty years after abortion was legalized, women have still not achieved pay equity in the workplace and they're still doing most of the work at home. Relying on contraception and abortion to plot and plan our families and futures has not been empowering for women.

It has been empowering for men.

*   *   *   *   *

Let's take a look back to the 1950s and 1960s, a time when I was growing up in Brooklyn. Most moms were "stay-at-home" moms. Mom cared for the children, did the shopping, laundry, cooking, and cleaned the home. The entire family ate a home cooked meal and sat around the kitchen table. They actually talked about their day. While it wasn't perfect, it provided a much more calm atmosphere than the "rat race" women find themselves in today.

While their number is shrinking, especially in our precarious economy, there are still some "stay-at-home" moms today and you might be wondering how they manage. Either they are fortunate enough to be well-situated financially or they have chosen to cut back on stuff. I can remember when I was raising my children in the 1980s, we had only one car and my daughters went to "Camp Mommy" in the summer. That meant they stayed home with me, with our small pool in the yard and summer activities that I planned.

In 2012, the financial investment web site Mint.com added up the things a stay-at-home mother does, and calculated what her salary would be if she were actually being paid: close to $100,000.

Imagine what a two-career Mom could make, first at her "real" job, and later, at her second shift gig at home— cooking, cleaning, doing the laundry, paying the bills, driving the kids to games and parties and the dentist.

In a way, I suppose you can say we do have it all, because very few doors remain closed to women. But the fact can't be overlooked that we are too tired, too drained, too spent to enjoy any of it very much. And the other fact that can't be overlooked is that, as of the end of 2012, 54 million unwanted, unplanned and "imperfect' children have been killed by abortion in the U.S.

Abortion doesn't empower women, it exploits them. It's bad medicine, bad morality, and even bad feminism.

Is this a major factor in our unhappiness? You bet it is!

Isn't it time to recall abortion?

CHAPTER SIX

"Well, I Had an Abortion and It Was Fabulous"

STATISTICS SHOW that one in ten American women will have an abortion by age twenty, one in four by age thirty, and one in three by age forty-five.[1] These statistics come from the Alan Guttmacher Institute, founded as the research arm for Planned Parenthood, the top abortion provider in the United States. Guttmacher and Planned Parenthood would like us to believe that most of these women are perfectly happy with their decision to abort.

Abortion providers, along with organizations like the National Organization for Women and NARAL, tell women that having an abortion is no big deal. You can have your abortion today and go back to school or work tomorrow. Your problem has been solved. Or has it?

We all know a woman who has had one or more abortions; I know thousands. Over the past two decades I have been involved with Rachel's Vineyard, Hope Alive, and Abortion Recovery International. These organizations deal directly with women (and fathers) who have had abortions, and it's through this involvement that I became aware of the devastating physical, psychological, and emotional impact of abortion.

Let's say after your abortion you are having trouble dealing with the fact that you terminated the life of your unborn child. Who do you tell? Where do you turn? It is very difficult to admit you have a problem with your abortion since it has been promoted as something good for women, a vital part of health care, and a constitutional right. Planned Parenthood and other "women's health" groups don't offer post-abortion counseling. They don't work to heal the physical and psychological scars. They merely get rid of a woman's baby in the name of choice, independence, and empowerment. So those feelings of regret, depression, and guilt get buried deep down inside. Many women struggle in silence for years, even decades.

While organizations like Rachel's Vineyard, Hope Alive, Abortion Recovery International, and my own Silent No More Awareness Campaign work to heal the wounds caused by abortion, and to give a voice to those who have suffered after having an abortion, groups like Planned Parenthood and NARAL attempt to whitewash the tragic consequences of abortion. It's ironic that a movement ostensibly concerned with choice, freedom, and empowerment, works so hard to silence its critics, even when those critics are *women* who had an abortion.

Consider the 2011 campaign on Twitter that asked women to say "I had an abortion," and to summarize that experience in 140 characters or less. The campaign was started by Steph Herold, a pro-abortion activist who launched the website IamDrTiller.com to honor the slain abortionist who killed children through the ninth month of their gestation. Through her Twitter campaign, Herold aimed to take away the stigma of abortion. One poster said the tweets also were a way to "silence" the men and women of Silent No More. But they will no longer be silent. Leave it to the pro-lifers (so often criticized for hating women) to actually give women a voice.

Many women regret their abortions, a fact that even the U.S. Supreme Court acknowledged in its 2007 decision, *Gonzales v. Carhart*: "The Act also recognizes that respect for human life finds an ultimate expression in a mother's love for her child. Whether to have an abortion requires a difficult and painful moral decision, which some women come to regret."[2]

Why is it then that the pro-abortion groups that claim to be the voice of the women in America, and that say "listen to the voices of women," won't acknowledge the voices of the women who regret their abortions? They would like them to remain silent about their regret, but these women want to reach out to those considering abortion and say, "Listen to our stories." Experience trumps rhetoric. So many women who now regret their abortion once had the same thoughts and feelings as the women who are considering abortion or the women who are tweeting that their abortion was a good decision. Eventually, one's true feelings rise to the surface. Abortion does not empower women. It causes the death of their child and—like it or not—a part of them also dies.

*   *   *   *   *

The last free-standing abortion clinic in Chattanooga, Tennessee, closed in 1993, and less than a year later, a pregnancy resource center was established at the site. The National Memorial for the Unborn was created on the other half of the property. Women who have aborted their babies can place a plaque with their child's name at the memorial. Visiting the memorial is a very powerful experience.

Kathryn B. drove six hundred miles and overcame an almost debilitating attack of nerves to be at the National Memorial for the Unborn in 2010 to tell the story of the choice she made nineteen years earlier to abort her baby.

"I actually believed the choice was somehow humane," said the Cleveland, Ohio, resident. "Like a lamb to the slaughter I signed the form."

What followed was self-recrimination and regret, inconsolable grief, unbearable guilt, and "a wound that would never heal."

After a time, Kathryn read *Forbidden Grief: The Unspoken Pain of Abortion*, co-authored by Rachel's Vineyard founder Dr. Theresa Karminski Burke. Kathryn finally found a way to forgive herself. Now she is one of more than nine thousand women and men who are part of the Silent No More Awareness Campaign. And she is one of hundreds who share their stories in public settings across the country, often with news cameras rolling, as they were that day in Tennessee.

"Women who have suffered the loss of their children by abortion are the victims of unspeakable trauma, a hideous unspoken violence," says Dr. Burke. "Why is it that Tweeters who claim to feel so empowered by abortion feel so intimidated and hyperaroused by the stories of other women who reveal the procedure as an emotionally wrenching act of destruction?"

In her work with the thousands of post-abortive women who come to Rachel's Vineyard retreats to be healed, Dr. Burke has seen how so many women have suffered in the aftermath of abortion.

No matter what your stance is on abortion, Burke says:

> It is important to accept the experiences of these women with tolerance and sympathy. They have something compelling to teach us about female oppression, discrimination, and a society that rejects women and the children of their wombs; about a planet where women are forced to be flattened in the name of freedom; about a tyranny which violates female instinct, femininity and women's unique role in procreation.

* * * * *

My colleague Dr. Alveda King, the niece of civil rights leader Martin Luther King Jr., leads the African–American outreach for Priests for Life and is an outspoken voice for Silent No More. She has also had two abortions, so she knows first-hand the pain of abortion, and she has seen how it cuts deeply into the African–American community. She has become one of the leading proponents for women's reproductive rights, which do not include the "right to choose."

"We should recognize that women become mothers the moment they are pregnant," Dr. King says. "The baby in the womb is a dependent, but fully human individual who is nourished and safeguarded by his or her mother. Any program that seeks to assist mothers should begin when motherhood begins, at pregnancy."

Dr. Burke agrees:

> True women's rights and freedom will never exist until our reproductive capacity is valued and the children we create are cherished by society and the men who father them. Violence against women will never end until society recognizes the benefits of fashioning life, instead of insisting upon its necessary destruction. So-called reproductive health by abortion is a counterfeit lie that threatens women and their children with violence and abandonment. The number one cause of death during pregnancy is murder. Abortion on demand has created a mindset that killing is the solution to unwanted responsibility—not just for the baby, but for the woman who won't exercise her "freedom of choice."

Like the women who came to the National Memorial for the Unborn in 2010 to place plaques with their baby's names on a memorial wall, Dr. King knows motherhood does not end with abortion.

"Women never forget the babies they gave up," she says, "no matter how compelling the reason seemed at the time." This is a far cry from the abortion industry's contention that abortion fixes a "problem," and afterwards life just continues on as before—or even better than before!

The "I Had an Abortion" campaign logged many posts from women who had not had abortions but want to keep their options open. Pro-lifers who posted opinions were sneered at by the pro-aborts, several of whom vowed that for every "anti-choice" post that popped up, they would donate money to an abortion fund.

Georgette Forney, president of Anglicans for Life and co-founder of Silent No More, added several tweets to the "I Had an Abortion Campaign" quoting women from the Silent No More Awareness Campaign.

She wrote that the campaign was "typical exploitation of women w/difficult choice. . . ." She referred other posters and those following the campaign to the free help available around the clock at Heartbeat International's Option Line that connects people to the pregnancy help network.

Unlike many of the posters who had no idea what it's really like to have made that choice, Mrs. Forney could say, "I Had an Abortion." And she, like countless others, will always regret it.

Let's hear from some more of the voices of the women of Silent No More. Leslie Graves of Wisconsin was pro-choice from an early age. She offered her testimony:

> I thought abortion was probably the right thing for a woman to do who wanted to achieve equality, have a career, and take advantage of her education. So, before I was ever in an unexpected pregnancy, I could

predict that I would choose an abortion.

As soon as I got pregnant when I was 20—I was in graduate school in philosophy—I immediately scheduled an abortion. It was a very physically safe abortion; there was a kind, caring staff, a clean, nice clinic. So it was certainly quite inexplicable to me why, two months later, I couldn't get out of bed in the morning because I was so depressed. I didn't understand why I ended up dropping out of graduate school later that semester. And I certainly didn't understand why, a few months later, I turned to my boyfriend with whom I had had the abortion and said, "You know, let's get married." And I chose as our wedding date the weekend that our child would have been due, because that was the only way that this still, small voice inside me that affirms life knew how to acknowledge and memorialize my child.

So as life went on I was still very pro-choice. I didn't know why I was starting to hate myself. I didn't know why, whenever I was pregnant again and I would be two and three months pregnant, I would wake up every morning and think that I probably should kill myself. I felt suicidal throughout my pregnancies. And when my babies were born, as much as I adored and loved them, I would wonder why I felt as if there was an invisible wall between us.

My experience is that this still, small voice we are all born with, that knows that life is sacred in spite of whatever ideologies we may embrace when we are young and foolish, is still there and speaks through us.

Leslie was pro-choice and chose abortion, and it took years for her to realize that her depression and difficulty bonding with her children were connected to her abortion.

Now let's look at another case. Debbie was sixteen when she had her abortion. Her mother, at the advice of a doctor, took Debbie to get the abortion. Her boyfriend and his parents, on the other hand, were making plans for this new life. When he discovered Debbie was going to abort the baby, he and his mother tried to persuade her not to. Debbie's mother intervened, and Debbie had the abortion. Immediately after the abortion, Debbie recalls:

> While in recovery I asked why I felt so sad. Would it go away? They told me it was relief from all the pressure that I had been under. They gave me something for pain and I fell asleep, crying. I woke up hurting and bleeding heavily. My mom was there. I heard girls crying. I started crying. I slept most of the way home. The abortion was never talked about again. It was like it never happened. . . . The abortion was supposed to fix everything, but it broke me instead. My body was never the same after the abortion.

Debbie ultimately married a man she met soon after her abortion, and they have three children. All three of her children were born prematurely, which she later learned was because of damage done to her cervix during the abortion. She also would have to undergo a total hysterectomy, which she attributes to the abortion. Debbie suffered physically from her abortion, but she also suffered psychologically:

With every pregnancy I went through, I saw my aborted baby in their eyes. I was full of wonder. I was also as pro-choice as you could be, very angry at the ones trying to tell women what they could or couldn't do with their own bodies. That anger and viewpoint validated my abortion. I had searched on the Internet for others who had had abortions.

I wondered if I was the only one hurting like this. I found Silent No More Awareness when it was just starting out. It was the first time I realized I wasn't alone. I wasn't crazy.

Debbie's story isn't the kind of testimony that Planned Parenthood or the "I Had an Abortion" campaign want you to hear. But Debbie is a real woman, who had a real abortion, and has experienced real suffering because of it.

The damage caused by abortion is not just physical, but psychological as well. The American Psychological Association, however, fails to acknowledge the many psychological problems that can occur after an abortion.

Cynthia Dillard had three abortions while she was studying for her degrees in clinical psychology. She has no clear memories of the first two abortions—the trauma has blurred her recall of the events. Ultimately she married the father of her aborted children, but looking back on that brief union that ended in divorce, she says, "that poor marriage, in a sense, was doomed from the beginning."

When she became pregnant a third time, with a new partner, she wanted to keep the baby but her boyfriend wanted her to have an abortion. "He was psychologically oppressive," she says. "Deep down I must have had some awareness of what I had done the first two times. Like many women who have had multiple abortions, there is a propensity to keep having abortions." And so she had the third.

As she continued her education, Cynthia began to experience anxiety and depression severe enough to require treatment. But never in her treatment, nor in her education, did the subject of abortion come up.

"It never occurred to me, despite extraordinary training . . . that my depression and anxiety was in any way related to my abortion. I never thought about it," she said. And because the academics and the psychology experts almost without fail were saying that abortion had no psychological impact on women, "I touted the party line," Cynthia says.

But after her third abortion, she says, "I began to question my value as a human in relation to God." That spiritual examination led her to the Catholic Church and to a new relationship with a man who also was converting to Catholicism and who she has since married. A Catholic friend in whom she confided about the abortions urged her to seek healing, and although she still didn't believe she had been damaged, she signed up for a Rachel's Vineyard retreat.

"I had a complete about-face," at the healing retreat, she said, "a 180-degree turn." She now knows that her anxiety and depression were the collateral damage of her abortions, and that there are millions of women suffering that same trauma.

Cynthia's story, and the others here, are just a small sampling of the many stories on the Silent No More website and I encourage you to read further about the devastation that abortion is causing to women, men, families, and society at large.

Isn't it time to recall abortion?

and in the fetal position in a room filled with other women who were all doing the same thing. I began to abuse drugs that I had never touched before. I did quite a bit of damage to myself. As time went on I felt angry, depressed, and hopeless. I began to obsess about my terrible deed, and felt I would surely go to hell for what I had done.

Christina undoubtedly suffers trauma as a result of her rape, but, clearly, she also suffers from the trauma of ending the life of her unborn child. Abortion did not alleviate her pain. It merely added new sufferings and more anguish.

Jody from Washington, D.C., offers a similar testimony:

My story begins many years ago when I was a young Army officer. I became pregnant as the result of a date rape. The choice I made to terminate that pregnancy would affect my life and ability to perform to my fullest potential as a soldier. I began to withdraw, isolate, suffer from anxiety, depression, sleep disorder, loss of self esteem, and a deep sense of loss. My overall mission as a soldier was compromised by the trauma I suffered as a result of that abortion. Later, I married another Army officer and eventually I left the military. However, I carried my baggage into my new life as an Army wife and eventually into motherhood. The daily routine of raising three active boys left little time to think about the past. When it did surface, I would suppress it and push it down into the deepest recesses of my mind. In due time, that suppressed memory came back and I could no longer shove it back into the box.

Again, abortion did not "solve" Jody's rape.

Nicole from Virginia also writes about how her abortion served only to make the trauma of her rape worse:

> I deeply regret the abortion I had four weeks after being raped. There is no good reason to have an abortion. All the logical reasons fail to keep your heart from breaking when it's over. If, like me, you were raped, and you think you can't bear nine months of pregnancy, I can tell you from experience the seventeen years of regret have been worse. I realized too late that my baby was a gift from a loving God who wanted to give me a purpose for my pain. . . . The abortion was the beginning of the real nightmare for me. . . . The abortion made healing from rape infinitely more difficult by compounding the trauma. . . . Abortion is not the answer for rape. It never was. But God is the answer for the pain.

Irene of the Netherlands was conceived when her father raped his wife. Her mother tried to commit suicide when she was six months pregnant but changed her mind. "I'm the face of someone who should not be here because of the way I was conceived," Irene said.

She did not know the circumstances of her conception when she herself became the victim of a violent rape, and later realized she was pregnant. In London, in a room with seven other women awaiting their turn to abort their "pregnancies," Irene had an epiphany, which she shared with a nurse. "I'm a mother," she remembers saying. "I have a child inside me." The nurse told her many women felt those last-minute jitters and reassured her she was doing the right thing. She remembers the abortionist being angry with her for slowing his assembly line. She also remembers the pain:

> When I came to, I was loudly told to stand. In agony I gripped my tummy with one hand, doubled with pain, while with the other I fumbled my way along the dark corridor wall, back to my bed in the other room. The other women were now silent and groaning with pain. My stomach felt as if every inch had been scraped open with a sharp razor blade. We were left alone . . . and after a long time . . . I believe the next day . . . I was allowed to go home, but the pain was unbearable. They offered a wheelchair, but I grit my teeth, saying to myself, "I wanted this, so grin and bear it." I bled profusely on the drive home, having to stop every now and then, dizzy, and was in absolute agony. The bleeding lasted half a year.

Once the bleeding stopped, Irene knew something else with certainty: "It wasn't the end of my problem." She suffered lumps in her breasts and complications with future pregnancies. She had trouble bonding with her future children. She acknowledged a simple and profound truth:

> I could have grown to love my child, just as my mother loved me. Life is not about how we were conceived, or our upbringing, but about what we make

of it. There is healing, and I am so glad my mother didn't have me killed when she had the chance. Pro-choice people might say I should have been murdered in the womb. I am so glad though that she gave birth to me, and raised me, despite how I was conceived, and that I am alive and able to now do something for humanity. My value and right to life does not depend on how I was conceived. Even after rape.

*   *   *   *   *

What about those women who were raped and decided to give birth? How did they feel? During their pregnancy were they reminded of the rape? Looking at their baby, did it remind them of the rapist? What about the child who was conceived as a result of rape? How do they feel when later they find out about their conception?

Liz was a seventeen-year-old high school student in Kentucky who was, in her own words, "always pro-life." But she had cause to question those convictions when she was drugged and date raped after a party during her senior year: "I would never have told anyone about it, except I got pregnant." She reasoned with herself that since the rape wasn't in any way her fault, she could get "an easy fix." She was still planning to have an abortion when a friend said to her, "you know you can't kill a baby."

Through Catholic Social Services she arranged an open adoption for the little boy who was born in the summer of 2007. People often ask her if she sees the face of her attacker when she looks at her son, who is being raised in a loving home. Her answer: "I have never seen anything other than that beautiful boy."

Juda's mother was walking home from a movie theater in St. Louis when she was gang-raped by eight men. When she learned she was pregnant, she decided over her mother's objections to offer the gift of life to her blameless child, and to make an adoption plan for her. Decades later, after learning the circumstances of her birth and adoption, Juda met her courageous birth mother. "It was the most wonderful reunion," she recalled. "She's a hero."

Although Juda was already pro-life, the knowledge that she was conceived in rape energized her pro-life activism. Juda has spoken at Harvard University, and both she and her mother have shared their story on television. Both have forgiven the rapist.

Juda knows that her mother was empowered by refusing to have an abortion. She went on to marry and have two more children. Now she also has two grandsons. To those pro-lifers who still believe that abortion should remain legal for rape victims, Juda says: "I am not the exception."

Cindy and her six younger siblings grew up in a Tennessee orphanage. When she was fourteen, their father showed up and moved them to Wisconsin. They settled in a crumbling, ancient house in a sparsely populated farming community. They were motherless as Cindy's mother had been found hanged in a basement in Memphis shortly after the birth of her seventh child.

In their strange new environment, their father was rarely home and when he was, she and her four sisters and two brothers would scatter in an effort to escape his abusive rage. "It was horrible," she recalled. "He would beat us all the time. We had no food and he kept a chain around the refrigerator with a padlock. He would go away a lot. We had no supervision at all."

The summer after she graduated from high school, Cindy was sleeping on a mattress on a floor in one of the upstairs bedrooms when a neighbor burst out of the closet and raped her.

"I had no idea what was happening. He had his way with me," she said. Cindy didn't even know the word rape, and she didn't know she had been the victim of a violent sexual crime. It was several months before she learned something else: she was pregnant.

People in the town saw her family as an unwelcome band of outsiders and some tried to shame Cindy into aborting her child. It was 1974 and abortion was legal throughout the country.

"When you come out of an orphanage, you don't know anything about the world, but I knew about abandonment," Cindy recalled. "People would abandon babies on our doorstep at the orphanage, and we loved those babies. I think God helped me realize that I couldn't abandon my own baby inside me. I understood that all little children are valuable."

With a Wisconsin winter closing in, Cindy's father flew into a rage and kicked her out of the house. She remembers her siblings crying and begging her not to leave them. "It struck me at that moment that I was homeless, motherless, penniless, and pregnant by rape," she said. "I went house to house in that town until

someone let me in and let me sleep on her couch."
She remembers with vivid clarity looking out the win-
dow of that temporary inn and seeing a bright winter
moon. She heard God speak these words to her: "This
daughter is sacred and of God. This child is destined
for great good." Cindy remembers thinking she didn't
know what "destined" meant but she knew aborting her
child would have been much worse than the rape she
endured.

She would spend the last few months of her pregnancy living with her mother's relatives, but her situation was not improved by much. Her room was in a
drafty basement and she was a virtual slave in their
home. When her daughter Jennifer was born, the family tried to take the baby away. Cindy escaped with her
three-moth-old daughter, found a tiny apartment over a
restaurant in Stillwater, Minnesota, and "learned what
welfare was." Cindy soon began a relationship with a man
who turned out to be "a spitting image of my father"—
an abusive drunk. They married and had a son, Jason.
After five years, Cindy had had enough, and found her
way to a Catholic church. A priest helped her secure an
annulment.

Years later, as an unmarried mother of two and a
devout Catholic, Cindy met Thomas, now her husband
of more than twenty-five years, at Mass. He adopted
Jennifer and Jason, and together the couple was able to
provide the stable, loving, happy family life that Cindy
had never experienced. "We broke the chain of the sins
of the father," she said.

Cindy's daughter Jennifer now has four children of

her own, and she has made good on the promise made to
Cindy that moonlit night in Wisconsin. She has worked
with war crimes victims in Bosnia and with children in
the notorious Romanian orphanages. She had a chance
to meet Pope John Paul II and she counsels women
against abortion.

Jennifer said that as she grew up and encountered
the argument, "We have to keep abortion legal because
of rape," she would simply tell people: "That is how I
came to be. I have been continually confirmed that God
has turned something awful into something redemptive,
as is His way, and that part of God's plan for me is to
change hearts just by simply being who He has created
me to be."

Cindy has forgiven her father and her rapist, and
has never regretted her decision to give birth to Jennifer. "The second Jennifer was born, nothing was on my
mind except the beautiful, dark-haired, blue-eyed baby
in my arms. I knew she was a gift. Her first smile, her
first tooth, her first word, these were healing for me. I
knew she was a gift."

*   *   *   *   *

Having an abortion allows the woman who has already
been so traumatized by rape to go through another
trauma. It punishes the innocent child. It punishes the
rape victim and mother. In fact, often the only person it
helps is the rapist, whose crimes are often covered up by
the abortion.

Now for the women who choose to have their baby

following the rape, the laws in many states *actually favor the rapist!*

Rebecca Kiessling was conceived by rape. She became a lawyer and works full-time to assist women who have been raped. "Having chosen life for her baby," said Ms. Kiessling, "now [the mother] has to make another choice."

The untold story of rape and abortion—another example of the real war against women—is what can happen to a woman once she chooses life for her baby following a rape. If the woman decides to prosecute the rapist, and his lawyer learns there is DNA evidence against him—that is, the baby—the rapist can sue for parental rights, visitation, and even custody. Often the rapist will only drop his claim on parental rights if the woman agrees not to prosecute.

Only eighteen states allow a judge to terminate a rapist's parental rights, and only one, Louisiana, mandates it. But in all eighteen states, a rapist has to first be convicted of rape. Ms. Kiessling pointed out that only about 1 percent of rapists are actually convicted of rape; the rest plead guilty to lesser charges. Some children of rape who are not aborted are being raised, at least part of the time, by the men who raped their mothers.

Another conundrum for a woman who keeps her baby after a rape is that if she applies for state aid to help her financially and names the rapist as the father, the state will go after him for financial support. If she had hoped never to see the rapist again and to keep her baby's existence a secret from him, that becomes impossible. On the other hand, if she doesn't name the rapist as the father, or can't because she doesn't know his identity, some states will cut off her funding, according to Ms. Kiessling.

Shauna Prewitt is an attorney who was raped, became pregnant, and chose to have and raise her daughter. What she discovered in her fight to keep her rapist away from her daughter was documented in a paper she wrote for the *Georgetown Law Journal*. Included in her findings was a mind-blowing double standard: Many states have streamlined the process for terminating a rapist's parental rights if the woman decides to make an adoption plan for her baby, but women who keep their babies find very little similar protection in the law.[2]

Furthermore, although the Hyde Amendment forbids that federal funds be used for abortions, abortions resulting from rape *can* be paid for with public funds. The government has made it easy to abort a child conceived in rape, and difficult to actually give birth. It sets up a situation where children conceived in rape begin life with fewer rights than anyone else, and their mothers, soon after experiencing the trauma of rape, are often encouraged to undergo further trauma.

When abortion is debated, whether in the media, in political races, or in private conversations, the argument for abortion in cases of rape seems to take center stage. You would think that there were huge numbers of abortions performed for this reason. But is that the reality?

No one has completely reliable numbers on the percentage of abortions that are performed because of rape, because not all rapes are reported and women might not reveal to an abortionist that rape is the reason they're aborting.

The Guttmacher Institute (founded as the research arm of Planned Parenthood) released a report in November 2012 on state abortion-reporting requirements. They found that only seven states require an abortionist to ask a woman if her pregnancy resulted from rape. That alone tells us that we don't really know what the exact figures are for women who abort because they became pregnant through rape.[3] Further, the Center for Disease Control, which produces the annual Abortion Surveillance reports, does not track the reasons why abortions are performed.

A study printed in 2000 by the American Journal of Preventive Medicine found that 333,000 sexual assaults and rapes were reported in 1998 and were responsible for 25,000 pregnancies.[4] An earlier study found about 30,000 rape-related pregnancies in 1996, with about half of them ending in abortion.[5]

In 2005, Guttmacher looked at two previous studies, one from 1987 and one from 2004, that asked women the reasons they were having abortions. In both studies, totaling just over 3,000 women, only 1 percent listed rape as a reason, and less than one half of 1 percent listed incest.[6]

While we don't have definitive numbers, it's clear from all these different indicators that the number of abortions performed each year for rape and incest victims is a very small fraction of the total number of abortions performed annually in the U.S. Despite its relative scarcity, abortions due to rape are often trumpeted by abortion supporters in an attempt to paint pro-lifers in a negative light.

Pro-abortion politicians, activists, and members of the media proclaim that the pro-life side hates women because we are against abortion even in cases of rape. But as we have shown, this is not the case. In fact, the opposite is true.

The testimonies of those conceived in rape and those who have become pregnant by rape show that abortion does nothing to erase the violence, fear, and trauma of the experience. In fact, for many women, abortion escalates their suffering.

When people ask pro-life advocates whether they oppose abortion even in cases of rape, they are really asking whether they care about the woman who has been victimized. Our answer is an unequivocal "Yes." Abortion helps neither the mother, who is traumatized again, nor the child, who is killed.

Isn't it time to love and protect them both? Isn't it time to recall abortion?

CHAPTER EIGHT

"I'm Against Abortion, but What About Fetal Anomalies?"

WHEN A baby in the womb is diagnosed with a life threatening or life-limiting disorder, many doctors—and well-meaning friends and relatives—will recommend abortion. But is an abortion a helpful solution in these cases? Let's look a little closer.

Several tests are performed during pregnancy to monitor the well-being of the unborn child. During the first trimester, routine blood tests and sonograms are performed. The number of sonograms depends upon the doctor. My daughter had a sonogram on every visit to her ob/gyn, every three weeks during the first and second trimester, and every week in the last trimester.

In the second trimester, most pregnant women have an alpha-fetoprotein (AFP) screening, a blood test that measures a protein normally produced by the fetal liver. Abnormal levels of AFP could mean the baby will be born with spina bifida, neural tube defects, Down syndrome, or other chromosomal abnormalities or defects. The test also can indicate twins, or a miscalculated due date. The AFP test, which is notorious for providing

false positives, is an indication that further, more inva-
sive testing is needed.

If a woman is older than thirty-five, amniocentesis
or chorionic villus sampling is recommended to look for
fetal anomalies. With many ob/gyns, once a patient has
a diagnosis of a fetal anomaly, termination of the pregnancy is discussed and in some cases strongly advised.
Let's look at some people who have had these experiences.

Laura Cuimei was pregnant with her second child
when her doctor sent her for an alpha-fetoprotein test
early in her second trimester. She and her husband Curt
were stunned when the results came back.

"They said I probably was carrying a Down syndrome
baby," the New Jersey resident recalled. "We were devastated. I was only 27 at the time and we never expected
something like that."

Her doctor was Catholic, working in a Catholic hospital, so he did not outright suggest that the couple consider abortion. "He dropped hints," Cuimei said. The
doctor did recommend amniocentesis, a prenatal diagnostic test in which a long needle is inserted through
a woman's stomach into the womb to draw up some of
the amniotic fluid surrounding the baby. The procedure,
although not very painful to the mother, carries a signifi-
cant risk of miscarriage. The Cuimeis declined.

"We knew that whether the baby had Down syndrome or not, we would love the baby," Mrs. Cuimei
said. A sonogram done a few weeks later indicated the
baby was fine, but the worry "was never far from my
mind." A full-term, healthy baby was born and the couple named him Christopher.

On Staten Island, Catherine Palmer had a similar situation with her first pregnancy. After spending eighteen months in a fertility clinic, undergoing several procedures and taking a variety of drugs, she and her husband Frank conceived through artificial insemination, which is when the man's sperm is injected directly into the uterus.

"Even before I got pregnant, doctors were warning me about the risk of multiple births with fertility drugs. That was the first time I ever heard the bone-chilling term 'selective reduction.' They were getting me used to the idea of abortion even before I was pregnant."

Finally pregnant, Catherine went to her regular ob/gyn, who sent her for the alpha-fetoprotein test at about fourteen weeks.

"I'll never forget this. The results came back showing the baby was at a high risk of both spina bifida and Down syndrome." The doctor recommended amnio, and the couple agreed, but they had to wait two weeks until Catherine's pregnancy was far enough along to perform the test. And then wait two more weeks for the results.

Four agonizing weeks later, her doctor called her at work with the results: a healthy baby boy was on his way.

"I will never forget the anxiety of those long weeks," Catherine said. "Before I got the results, I had already begun to feel him move. There's no way I would have aborted that baby, but the attitude I encountered a lot of different places along the way was that it would be better to abort and try again.

"Good thing we didn't!"

While both Laura and Catherine said they would not have aborted their Down syndrome babies, the shocking truth is that a majority of couples—up to 90 percent, according to some studies—choose to abort after receiving a prenatal diagnosis of Down syndrome.

Another disease that is diagnosed in utero is Cystic Fibrosis (CF). I interviewed Kristan Hawkins, a mom who has a child with Cystic Fibrosis. Here's what Kristan had to say:

> I had never heard the term cystic fibrosis until I was pregnant with my first son, Gunner. I remember the physician's office asking me whether or not I wanted to undergo a prenatal screening for the disease. I didn't know what CF was but like with Down Syndrome, I chose not to have any prenatal screening tests performed as I knew no matter how Gunner was born my husband and I would love him unconditionally, and I was not willing to take the chance that the test could cause me to miscarry.
>
> Gunner's birth on January 30, 2009 was normal, as normal as any birth goes, and his Apgar score was great. All was well in the world. For two weeks, my husband and I were on "cloud 9." Then Gunner's pediatrician called us and asked us to bring Gunner in to re-do one of his newborn screening tests and to alert us that Gunner was not gaining weight. After the score for one of the CF marker tests came back positive, we were scheduled for a sweat test on St. Patrick's Day. Sweat tests are simple procedures that can, in most circumstances, actually predict whether

or not an individual has CF. The couple of weeks leading up to the test, my husband and I read everything we could about cystic fibrosis and the devastating disease that it can be. We were scared, scared for our son and scared for our family—how would we take care of him and afford all of his medical needs. I remember the night before the test, waking up as my husband was crying in bed with Gunner laying next to him saying, "He has it. He has it. He tastes salty." Those with CF have high salt deposits in their sweat.

The next morning, we took Gunner to the hospital for the test and within hours Gunner's pediatrician called to confirm that Gunner has CF. Our world, the perfect world that my husband and I had envisioned for our family, was gone in an instant. Everything had changed.

Over the next few months, our number one goal was getting Gunner healthy, into the best hospitals, and on the right medications. But during that time, the national debate regarding the newly sworn-in President Obama's national health-care plan, an issue that quite frankly previously bored me before, began raising alarms. I started hearing and reading terms that got me wondering, what would happen in a state-run health-care system to those like Gunner, preborn and born. What I found while researching was shocking. Just like with Down Syndrome, 90 percent of children diagnosed with CF during pregnancy are aborted. And those who President Obama appointed to high-levels of his cabinet and were publicly acknowledged as authors of his plan, Obamacare, had some very alarming things to say about those who require the most medical assistance. Those like Dr. Donald Berwick who was appointed to the Department of Health and Human Services to oversee the nation's Medicaid and Medicare system who had worked with Great Britain's National Health Service (NHS) to re-make their current nationalized health care system, which rations care to those who need it most each year. Berwick was even on record openly acknowledging that health care rationing occurs and that the state must determine if additional treatments/medications to certain citizens are of value to the taxpayers or if funds could be better used.

After organizing several coalition efforts with parents of children with other genetic disease like Down Syndrome and Trisomy 18 for the past two years, I can honestly say that we have a long way to go. While I truly believe we are winning the hearts and minds of Americans on the issue of abortion, we are losing on the issues of embryonic personhood and prenatal screening.

Today in America, women who receive a positive result for their preborn child during a Down Syndrome or cystic fibrosis test widely report they are pressured to abort. In IVF procedures, it is common and standard care to "screen out" any embryos with these diseases. When was I pregnant with my second son, Bear, I was asked on multiple occasions if I wanted to test him for hereditary cystic fibrosis and, then after his healthy delivery, I was offered multiple times to have a contraceptive device implanted in me to prevent me from getting pregnant again, while I was still under the influence of painkillers.

Already, ethicists here in America and abroad are calling for increased and government-mandated genetic tests to be performed on every mother, so as to encourage any family with a positive result *(which we know can be, at times, false)* to abort and try again for a 'better' baby. Some of these "ethicists" are even calling it the morally responsible thing to do. It's harder to find statistics on other disorders that are diagnosed in utero, but even without hard numbers, it's crystal clear where *Roe v. Wade* has led us in 40 years. It seems we have decided, as a society, that if babies are not perfect, they don't deserve to live.

Where fetal anomalies or illness is involved, it has increasingly become the case that abortion is recommended and even encouraged.

*   *   *   *   *

According to Dr. Mary Davenport, an ob/gyn in California, the American College of Obstetricians and Gynecologists (ACOG) was against abortion in the 1950s and early 1960s. But by the late 1960s, when the birth control pill was growing in popularity, things changed.

"When the Supreme Court made its *Roe v. Wade* decision, ACOG applauded," Dr. Davenport said. "But the membership never voted on it. The elite people at the top, who were aligned with Planned Parenthood, made a policy decision that abortion was an advance in women's health."

In 1993, ACOG published a "College Statement of Policy" on abortion that has been reaffirmed repeatedly, most recently in 2011. It reads: "ACOG supports access to care for all individuals, irrespective of financial status, and supports the availability of all reproductive options. ACOG opposes unnecessary regulations that limit or delay access to care."[1]

In an opinion paper on conscientious refusal published in November 2007, ACOG wrote that those physicians who do not want to perform abortions for religious, ethical, or moral reasons should set up shop close to abortionists, or at least be willing to refer patients for abortions.[2] Dr. Davenport said pro-life physicians agree that this recommendation makes conscience rights practically a moot point.

To add a pro-life voice to the increasingly pro-abortion dialogue, Dr. Matt Bulfin founded an organization within ACOG shortly after *Roe v. Wade*. His group, the American Association of Pro-Life Obstetrician-Gynecologists (AAPLOG), has been "a thorn in the side" of the main organization ever since, said Dr. Davenport, who is now president of AAPLOG.

While AAPLOG has indeed been a thorn in the side of the medical community, the fact remains that the overarching policy of ACOG is to recommend abortion in cases of fetal anomalies. It is a despicable practice, often predicated upon unreliable information. All life is precious, and all babies deserve to live. And those babies who have anomalies or illnesses are no exception.

*   *   *   *   *

So you might be asking, what about those couples who went with a doctor's advice to terminate the pregnancy? How did they feel afterward?

Nancy Kreuzer from Illinois writes:

> I was five and a half months pregnant when I was told that she [my baby] had water on the brain (hydrocephalus) and was advised by my doctor to "terminate the pregnancy." It was explained that the abortion would be a simple procedure. My husband and I were told we could leave this behind us, get on with our lives and try for another baby.
>
> Because I was in my second trimester of pregnancy, the abortion was a two-day procedure. It was not, as the doctor described, "simple." At the abortion clinic no one asked how I was or explained what was happening to me. I felt alone, afraid and devastated. While I sat, waiting for the doctor to arrive, many nurses and workers in the abortion clinic casually walked by me. I sat there for hours. Tears streamed down my face but no one talked to me, no one acknowledged my pain.
>
> The day after my abortion, I felt numb. I left the abortion clinic with no baby to bury, no doll-size casket, no funeral service, no grave to adorn with flowers. I vomited in the parking lot and rode home in silence. No one brought meals, no one sent cards, no one called, because I had been too ashamed to tell anyone what I had agreed to. In the weeks to follow,

I tried to bury the memory of the abortion and not look back.

In the months and years afterward, there were clear signs that the scars of my abortion existed, but I didn't recognize them at the time. Interestingly, I assumed I was doing just fine. But below the surface, I was unusually fearful. As time went on, I often had the sense that I wanted to run and I had repeated nightmares of running from something horrible. I would awaken panicked, unable to sleep the rest of the night. There was an internal sadness, not visible to the world.

When these heartbreaking situations arise in pregnancy, when a couple learns their child has an illness that will end his or her life days or minutes after birth, what are their options? Because abortion is legal throughout pregnancy, couples often choose to abort these late-term babies because they are led to believe by their doctors that they have no other choice.

"In medicine, children are looked at as sexually transmitted diseases," said Dr. John Bruchalski, who performed abortions as part of his medical residency in obstetrics and gynecology. He said that at the time, he believed contraception and abortion were necessary "in order to bring women health and happiness."

Following a "radical awakening," the Virginia resident and member of ACOG stopped doing abortions and months later also stopped prescribing contraception.

"We've always been taught in ob/gyn that we have two patients, that there are two lives there," said Dr.

Davenport. "But now people are told really ridiculous things about needing to abort their babies that are not even true."

But why would physicians, particularly those who have chosen obstetrics as a specialty, be so quick to suggest abortion? According to Dr. Davenport and Dr. John Bruchalski, doctors who are already paying high malpractice insurance are afraid of being sued for "wrongful birth" if babies are born any less than perfect.

"Ninety-five percent of all doctors in the U.S. will recommend abortion," if babies are found to have any of a growing list of diseases or disorders, Dr. Bruchalski said. "We have become eugenicists overnight."

Dr. Davenport said doctors insist on pre-natal testing under the guise of giving their patients time to prepare for the challenges of dealing with a sick child. But that's a ruse, she said. "They can be liable for a lot of money. That's the bottom line. It's given so many doctors a eugenic orientation."

Birth defects once were considered unexpected setbacks, challenges for parents who assumed they would be coming home from the hospital with a perfect baby girl or boy. But in our abortion-friendly, litigious society, birth defects have become actionable offenses.

A wrongful birth suit, recognized in forty-five states, is brought by parents who assert they would have aborted had they known their baby would be born with a serious illness. Wrongful life, recognized only in four states (California, New Jersey, Maine, and Washington), is brought on behalf of an infant and claims it would have been better had he or she never been born. This is not the stuff of science fiction; this is real and happening now.

In "Burdened By Life," a commentary in the March 2011 edition of the *Albany Government Law Review*, attorney Brady Begeal argued against this callous disregard for life:

> Parents undoubtedly face daunting emotional and financial burdens when they raise a child who has a disability. However, allowing an action for wrongful birth or wrongful life is not the answer. These claims encourage eugenic abortions, by both parents and by medical providers alike. For someone who is actually living life with a disability, recognition of these causes-of-action must seem disrespectful and morally reprehensible, if not utterly revolting. While many courts and state legislatures, like New York, have limited the damages that can be sought by plaintiffs, this is not enough. Instead, state legislatures should reevaluate this line of prenatal torts, and send a message that respects those living with disabilities, and encourages life. Alternative routes of compensation for parents, such as increased funding for those parents so that out-of-pocket expenses are minimized, should be considered. Such an approach would be a better public policy alternative than permitting lawsuits that carry significant eugenic and discriminatory implications.[3]

Is there an alternative to abortion and wrongful life suits? Absolutely.

With the proliferation of perinatal (the word mean "means around the time of birth") hospice programs across the country during the last ten years, couples with a dire perinatal diagnosis do have a choice, one that allows their baby to be loved and cherished for as long as he or she survives. It's a better choice than abortion for everyone, according to Dr. Byron Calhoun, one of the pioneers of the perinatal hospice movement.

"We had to have something to offer people other than 'don't do that,'" Dr. Calhoun said of late-term abortions. He and a colleague began discussing the need for a compassionate option during the mid-1990s, when the nation was embroiled in the partial-birth abortion debate. Until that time, no one gave much thought to late-term abortion or the brutal and inhumane ways these nearly born children are killed. Partial-birth abortion is largely banned now, but as an alternative to that barbaric practice, many late-term abortions now are accomplished by the equally barbaric method of dismembering the babies while they are still in the womb.

When he was still performing abortions, Dr. Bruchalski realized the truth about this procedure. "When you kill another human life up close and personal, it's viciously brutal," he said. "The baby fights back a little bit. When they get real big, they don't want to be killed."

The alternative to this soul-scarring procedure is perinatal hospice. Parents are able to plan for the birth with the support of doctors, nurses, counselors, clergy, and family. Babies are bathed, dressed, cuddled, and surrounded by the love every baby deserves, and when they die, it is with the dignity every human being deserves. Parents who choose perinatal hospice still have to deal with the grief that comes from losing a child, but studies have shown they can deal with that grief much better than women who choose late-term abortion.

"We explain that they're not going to escape any of the grief, but we ask them if they want to spend time with their babies," Dr. Calhoun said, adding that 75 percent of couples choose perinatal hospice when it's offered.

For those who are able to nurture and cherish their infants, "there's grief and there's sadness," Dr. Calhoun said. "But there's no post-traumatic stress."

*   *   *   *   *

There was never any doubt that Paulina and Matt Rudman would choose a short life over a brutal death for their conjoined twins. By choosing life, Paulina is convinced, her own life was saved.

Immediately after giving birth to the premature girls in 2007, Paulina's blood pressure plummeted, and doctors worried she wouldn't make it. She already had seven children, and all but one of them was there in the Ohio hospital with her and her husband to be part of the extraordinary birth. The babies, Lucija and Mija, were conjoined twins whose two brains shared a skull. Their hearts were fused and they were born in an embrace that carried them to heaven just ninety minutes later.

As Paulina's life was slipping away, she looked at the just-baptized girls cradled in the arms of their father and said, "I walked a thousand miles for you, and now you have got to help me pull through this."

Paulina's "thousand miles" began not quite four

months earlier, on January 22, 2007, when she learned the baby she'd been carrying for twelve weeks had a chromosomal defect and such severe abnormalities that a doctor, after viewing her ultrasound, told Mrs. Rudman she would miscarry in a week or two. A month later she was back in his office, where he was mystified to find the baby's heart still beating.

In between doctor visits, her youngest daughter, then two, learned she was about to become a big sister. She got strangely quiet after hearing the news, and then pronounced that the baby was a girl and her name was Lucy. Paulina agreed to name her Lucija if she was indeed a girl. She announced her plans to the doctor at her second visit. "He thought we were crazy," she recalled. He sent her home to await her miscarriage. Initially she and her husband kept the baby's condition to themselves but at this point they were ready to share the news. "She's here now," Paulina said. "She might not be here tomorrow, but I want everyone to know she's here now."

By the end of April, Paulina was sixth months pregnant. "I was huge," she said. "I could barely move. I felt like I was full-term." Another ultra-sound was suggested, and its results were even more startling than the first. There was not one baby, but two. The way they were joined explained many of the abnormalities discovered on the earlier ultrasounds, but it didn't change their prognosis. One of Paulina's first thoughts was that they would need a second name. "We named her Mija, because it was the first of May."

A meeting was scheduled to decide how to proceed. The Rudmans brought Dr. Andrew True, a bioethicist, with them. "Any decision we made had to be in keeping with the teachings of the Church." Her only wish was that she could deliver the babies alive and that they would live long enough to be baptized into the Catholic faith that had always sustained their family. The girls were expected to live no longer than fifteen minutes. It would be a race against time. Paulina insisted on a C-section to maximize the chances the girls would be born alive.

Before her scheduled C-section, she found herself "going to the funeral home picking out a casket, knowing my baby girls were alive. What was surreal had become bizarre." And yet somehow, she was able to still feel joy, knowing there was life inside her.

Mija and Lucija were born May 13, 2007, the Feast of Our Lady of Fatima, when Mary appeared to three children in Portugal, including a young girl named Lucia. Together the girls weighed three pounds, four ounces. A priest was with them at the birth and, as doctors stitched Paulina up, he whisked the babies and the rest of the Rudmans away so the babies could be baptized. A photographer was on hand. Everyone had a chance to hold the girls. Days later, five priests concelebrated their funeral mass.

"They were really quite beautiful in their own way," Paulina said. "God let us see something through His eyes, to be able to behold something that was hideous and see the beauty. Jesus said, 'I and the Father are one and the same, one mind, one heart.' They truly were created in the image of God."

Paulina pulled through and has never looked back with regret. "I had such peace, such a grace that came to us after. I was so whole after, more whole than I had ever been in my life. The grace of doing what was right even though it was hard was astounding to me."

*   *   *   *   *

A 2002 story in *The Leaven*, a Catholic newspaper in Kansas City, Kansas, told the story of Nancy Stanfield. Early in her second trimester, it was determined that her baby had an open neural tube defect. It causes the skull to stop growing and leaves the brain exposed and undeveloped. Their doctor told them their options would be to be induced at five months or to have a partial-birth abortion. The Stanfields, shocked at even the suggestion of abortion, chose the induction, but Nancy's water broke three weeks before the scheduled delivery date. But the Stanfields had already made plans for a priest to be on hand. Reporter Bethanne Scholl wrote:

> When the C-section was concluded, the surgical team saw the priest standing outside the door, and they motioned him in. "They had a little blanket and wrapped it around the baby and brought him around to Nancy," said the priest. "I went right to her and anointed her, and then I got the holy water and baptized the baby." "He stopped breathing then, but his heart continued to beat." Nancy believes that was the moment Colby left them.
>
> "I cried out loud, 'Mama loves you, Colby . . . Mama loves you,'" said Nancy.
>
> After months of fearing the worst, Nancy looked

at her baby boy, bruised from the C-section and minus the baby fat of a full-term baby. And she fell in love. "Our first son, Brady, was bald for so long," said Nancy. "Colby had dark hair across the top of his forehead, where his hairline would have started."

The Stanfields marveled at their newborn. "I hardly cried that day," said Nancy. "We were really unprepared for how happy that day was. I felt so good. We couldn't see doing it any other way."

When Nancy was first trying to convince a family member that the decision to carry Colby was the right one, he told her she was only doing it because she had become a Catholic. "I told him that wasn't true," said Nancy. "Even if I hadn't become a Catholic, I would have made this decision. It isn't a Catholic decision. It's a human one."[4]

As Nancy said, her decision was not about faith, it was a human decision. The problem is that as a society we have allowed abortion to enter into our midst, which has permitted us to look at children as commodities. Also parents feel entitled to a perfect child. I can remember back in 1978 when I was expecting my first child and sonograms weren't even in use, you waited with wonderment. Was the baby a girl or a boy? We all prayed for a healthy baby; ten fingers and ten toes was the phrase we used back then. Even though abortion was legal, medical science had not aggressively started down the road to all those prenatal tests. I remember when my daughter was born, the woman in the bed next to me had a baby boy born with a cleft lip and palate. I remember all the specialists coming to prepare her for what would lie ahead—multiple surgeries, physical and speech therapy. What might the fate of that baby boy been today? He might well have become another abortion statistic.

There are alternatives, and help, for parents facing a pregnancy with a fatal or abnormal diagnosis. Organizations like Prenatal Partners for Life are dedicated to providing families—those who have or are expecting a special-needs child—the support, information and encouragement they need to make informed decisions involving their preborn or newborn child's care. They believe these children are unique gifts from God and have a special purpose in life that only they can fulfill. Their goal is to provide honest, practical information about parenting a special-needs child by linking expectant parents or new parents with those who are already caring for these cherished children.*

And don't forget the perinatal hospice programs pioneered by Dr. Bryon Calhoun. Perinatal hospice and palliative care are innovative and compassionate models of support that can be offered to parents who find out during pregnancy that their baby has a life-limiting condition. As prenatal testing continues to advance, more families are finding themselves in this heart-breaking situation. Perinatal hospice incorporates the philosophy and expertise of hospice and palliative care for terminally ill adults for this new population of tiny patients. For parents who receive a life-limiting prenatal diagnosis and

---

* Visit www.prenatalpartnersforlife.org to learn more about the organization.

wish to continue their pregnancies, perinatal palliative care helps them embrace whatever life their baby might have, before and after birth. These programs are growing around the country and the world. You can find locations and more information at www.perinatalhospice.org.

I also recommend the website www.BeNotAfraid. net where parents in these situations have an opportunity for discussion and support.

After reading just a handful of testimonies from parents who aborted their children after an abnormal or fatal diagnosis and learning about their on-going trauma and regret, and comparing their experiences to those of parents who chose life for their children, wouldn't you agree it's time to recall abortion?

CHAPTER NINE

"I'm Against Abortion, but What About the Life of the Mother?"

DURING A November 2011 debate in the House of Representatives over a bill that would have stopped abortion funding and enhanced conscience rights in the Affordable Care Act (a.k.a. Obamacare), former House Speaker Nancy Pelosi claimed the bill would allow doctors to let women "die on the floor" of emergency rooms because they could refuse to perform an abortion even if the woman's life depended on it.

Nothing of the sort would have happened had the bill passed. But that bit of theater on Capitol Hill served as a good demonstration of just how misunderstood the position of the pro-life movement in general, and the Catholic Church in particular, is when it comes to a pregnancy that endangers the life of the mother.

According to the teachings of the Catholic Church, a doctor cannot abort a child to save the mother. If the child dies during a life-saving procedure or treatment for the mother, the unborn baby's death is an unfortunate but unavoidable side effect. To try to save them both, doctors will allow the pregnancy to progress as long as possible without jeopardizing the mother, then deliver the baby and do everything possible to keep the child alive. Some call it a waste of money. I call it good medicine. Remember the Hippocratic Oath: "First, do no harm."

"It's always wrong to directly kill an innocent human being, regardless of their stage of life," said Dr. John Haas, president of the National Catholic Bioethics Center in Philadelphia. "If you make a list of exceptions, where does it stop? There's no logical place to draw that line. All human life is sacred, and has to be sacred."

The way the issue is presented in the mainstream media, however, gives the impression that mothers have to choose between their lives and their babies' lives every day, and that there is widespread agreement that the mother's life always prevails.

"Given the entrenched power of the cultural elite in this country," Haas said, "it will take a miracle . . . to bring about a change in the way we have come to view the unborn."

"We hit the bottom of the slippery slope in this country in 1973, when it became legal for private citizens to take the lives of other private citizens," he said. "In principle, it can't be any worse than that."

But pro-life physicians like Dr. John Bruchalski, founder of the Tepeyac Family Center in Virginia, have come to a different understanding.

"You never pit the life of the mother against the life of the child, but given our abortion-friendly culture," Bruchalski said, doctors sometimes find themselves "encouraging heroism" in mothers whose pregnancies might put them at risk and who might lean toward abortion before having all the information they need.

"You have to have a relationship with the patient to be able to convince her that you won't let her die and that her baby doesn't have to die either," Bruchalski said. "What we do with mothers at risk is practice good medicine. We monitor her, in the hospital or even in intensive care if we need to. We deliver the baby when we have to."

Since he began a private practice in 1991, he has never had an at-risk mother die.

Many doctors will recommend abortion for women suffering from heroin withdrawal, cardiomyopathy, hypertension, or aortic stenosis. Many physicians will insist on abortion for women with pulmonary hypertension or severe lupus. For these women, Dr. Bruchalski said, it might become necessary to deliver their babies before they are viable, leaving those babies with a high probability of death. But delivering a baby is a far cry from aborting a baby, as the American Association of Pro-Life Obstetrician Gynecologists notes in it official policy statement:

> Abortion is the purposeful killing of the unborn in the termination of a pregnancy. AAPLOG opposes abortion. When extreme medical emergencies that threaten the life of the mother arise (chorioamnionitis or HELLP syndrome could be examples), AAPLOG believes in "treatment to save the mother's life," including premature delivery if that is indicated—obviously

with the patient's informed consent. This is NOT "abortion to save the mother's life." We are treating two patients, the mother and the baby, and every reasonable attempt to save the baby's life would also be a part of our medical intervention. We acknowledge that, in some such instances, the baby would be too premature to survive.[1]

Dr. Byron Calhoun, a pioneer in prenatal hospice, said physicians "just need to be doctors. Control the diabetes. Control the hypertension. Treat your patient. You don't have to kill the baby. It's a ridiculous argument to justify killing a baby."

Dr. Calhoun said there have been only three or so times during his years in practice that he has had to deliver a baby before twenty-four weeks. About 50 percent of babies born in the twenty-fifth or twenty-sixth week will survive. That rate goes up to 90 percent for babies who can stay in the womb until twenty-eight weeks. Dr. Calhoun offers sage advice to other physicians: "Just be a doctor and treat two patients, the mother and her unborn child."

*   *   *   *   *

You can imagine the psychological toll it takes on women who abort their child to avoid health risks or possible death. Not only does abortion "to save the life of the mother" kill a child—like all abortions—it can also have severe emotional effects on the mother.

Here's the story of one woman who took her doctor's

advice and ended the life of her unborn child because she was led to believe her life was in jeopardy.

Cheryl from California was born with a defective aortic valve and it played a role in the birth of her first child:

> After I gave birth to my daughter Stephanie, I could not breathe but the heart doctor thought I would make it. When I got pregnant again, I was so weak I could not care for my other two children. By now I knew the Lord well but my faith left me and fear haunted my every step.
>
> Everyone I spoke to said that I had two other children to care for and it was all right if I chose my life over the life of my unborn baby. Oh this haunted me. I just wanted to die. What kind of mother puts her life before that of her unborn child? No one that I spoke with ever counseled me. It took me years to forgive myself. Now I realized I was not more important than my unborn child. Oh how many nights I was in total depression and did not know why because I was not allowed to speak of it, except when I told a friend of my guilty secret.
>
> My husband hated me for doing this, so when he would drink he called me horrible names in front of our other children. But I knew I deserved that and more. One day God healed me of that brokenness and I promised him never to lose the sanctity of life again.

Cheryl's experience confirms what so many other women have said in the testimonies you've read. For many women, having an abortion leaves lifelong psychological scars. A mother's maternal instinct is to save her child. What mother on a sinking ship would not put the life vest on her children first? If a car was careening out of control, wouldn't every mother push the baby carriage out of the way first, even if that meant she might be hit by a car?

Lyndsey Crowder, for one, decided to have her baby even though her life was in severe danger. Her story was published by England's *Daily Mail.*

Ms. Crowder and her husband had already suffered a stillbirth and the miscarriage of twins when they found out she was pregnant again. A few weeks later, she was diagnosed with Hodgkins lymphoma and was told she might only have weeks to live.

Ms. Crowder told a reporter for the *Daily Mail* that "to my mind, there was no choice. I knew I had to give the baby a chance." The newspaper reported that the thirty-four-year-old had a tumor the size of a small football in her chest when she began eight rounds of chemotherapy. She delivered a healthy baby girl by C-section at thirty-four weeks, and then went on to have a bone marrow transplant and radiation treatments. She is now in remission and her daughter, Sidney Rose, is healthy. She recalled that when she first received the diagnosis, she realized, "I can deal with the cancer but I cannot lose another baby." [2]

The following is an excerpt from a story by Peter Baklinski that was published by Lifesite News in November 2011.

on *Today*, she was a healthy five-month-old, right where she was supposed to be developmentally. Linsey was on the road to remission.

Linsey and Lena's story highlights the importance of finding doctors who don't immediately leap to the abortion conclusion when presented with any kind of obstacle during a pregnancy. A pro-abortion doctor might well have scared Linsey with a terrible prognosis of her own chances, and reassured her that she could "try again" once she was well. But she wouldn't have had Lena, and she would have carried the burden of knowing her survival came at the cost of her daughter's life.

Choosing life is always the right choice, even when it's hard, even when it's scary, even when the outcome is unclear. And given advances in medicine in the past decades, the so-called choice between baby and mother is becoming increasingly rare, even to the point that it is practically nonexistent.

A 1996 piece published in *First Things* by Dr. Thomas Murphy Goodwin, then the director of maternal-fetal medicine at Good Samaritan Hospital in Los Angeles, shed some much-needed light on how rare it is to find a woman whose life is actually threatened by her pregnancy:

> My practice and clinical research are in a sub-specialty of obstetrics and gynecology, maternal-fetal medicine, which concerns pregnancies complicated by maternal or fetal disease. There are few situations more daunting to those who advocate a consistent ethic of life than the circumstance in which the life of the mother

is threatened by the continuation of the pregnancy. Although I do not acknowledge this conflict as justifying abortion, even the most dedicated of advocates for the life of the unborn are awed by this dilemma. Indeed, the power of this image has been one of the principal forces advancing the abortion movement in the United States and elsewhere. What do we know about it objectively?

Certain conditions that can be diagnosed in advance are associated with risk of maternal mortality greater than 20 percent: pulmonary hypertension (primary or Eisenmenger's syndrome), Marfan's syndrome with aortic root involvement, complicated coarctation of the aorta, and, possibly, peripartum cardiomyopathy with residual dysfunction. Taken altogether, abortions performed for these conditions make up a barely calculable fraction of the total abortions performed in the United States, but they are extremely important because they have been used to validate the idea of abortion as a whole. They stand as a sign that abortion is in some cases unavoidable—that it can be the fulfillment of the good and natural desire of the mother to live.

It should be emphasized how rare these conditions are. Our obstetric service in the Los Angeles area has been the largest in the United States for most of the last fifteen years, averaging fifteen thousand to sixteen thousand births per year. Our institution serves a catchment for all high-risk deliveries in an area with thirty thousand deliveries per year. Excluding cases that have been diagnosed late in pregnancy, we do not see more than one or two cases per year that pose this degree of risk of maternal mortality; these are exceedingly rare conditions. This rarity does not diminish the tragic dimension of such cases, but the cases are seen in perspective when their numbers are compared to the total number of abortions performed.[4]

As Dr. Goodwin points out, even though they are extremely rare, there are still cases where both the life of the baby and the life of the mother hang in the balance.

Those who advocate for abortion often fall back on the example of ectopic pregnancy to show how women's lives would be in danger if abortion became illegal again. In an ectopic pregnancy, a fetus begins to develop outside the womb, most often in a fallopian tube. This is almost always a non-viable pregnancy, and it carries a high risk of rupture of the tube, which can kill the mother. No physician would refuse to treat a mother in such a circumstance. But doctors and couples who adhere to a "no exception" policy on abortion, and are faithful to the teachings of the Catholic Church, must be careful in choosing their method of treatment.

The United States Conference of Catholic Bishops, in its 2009 update of its "Ethical and Religious Directives for Catholic Health Care Providers" was unambiguous about acceptable treatment for ectopic pregnancy: In case of extrauterine pregnancy, no intervention is morally licit which constitutes a direct abortion.

There are several ways to treat ectopic pregnancy, and some of them do constitute a direct abortion.

Treatment with the miscarriage-inducing Methotrexate, and a surgical procedure that directly removes the embryo through an incision in the wall of the fallopian tube are becoming more common because they are more likely to preserve the fallopian tube, which means a woman has a better chance of conceiving again. But make no mistake, both of these methods are direct abortions.

Another method of treatment for an ectopic pregnancy is the salpingectomy, which removes all of the tube, or just the part where the embryo is attached. According to Catholics United for the Faith, most Catholic theologians say the salpingectomy is morally acceptable:

> A partial salpingectomy is performed by cutting out the compromised area of the tube (the tissue to which the embryo is attached). The tube is then closed in the hope that it will function properly again. A full salpingectomy is performed when implantation and growth has damaged the tube too greatly or if the tube has ruptured. These moralists maintain that, unlike the first two treatments, when a salpingectomy is performed, the embryo is not directly attacked. Instead, they see the tissue of the tube where the embryo is attached as compromised or infected. The infected tube is the object of the treatment and the death of the child is indirect. Since the child's death is not intended, but an unavoidable secondary effect of a necessary procedure, the principle of double effect applies. . . . [5]

A direct abortion is very rarely, if ever, a medical necessity, and it is *never* morally right. Furthermore, we have seen the effects these decisions have on the mother. The psychological trauma is often great. These mothers will spend the rest of their lives with the knowledge that they sacrificed their child's life for their own well being.

And yet "life of the mother" is one of the most commonly heard rallying cries of the pro-abortion movement. Less than 3 percent of the more than one million abortions performed annually are done as a result of rape, incest, fetal anomaly, or life of the mother. We know from reading the experiences of those who chose life even in these hard cases that there are always options.

Isn't it time we stop justifying murder? Isn't it time to recall abortion?

CHAPTER TEN

A Hard Pill to Swallow

SO FAR, we've covered abortion in all different types of circumstances, and for a myriad of reasons. We've read the testimonies of women who have had abortions, and the testimonies of women who decided not to have abortions. One thing is for certain, abortion kills an unborn child and it harms women, mentally, physically, and psychologically.

While many people consider abortion to be wrong, many of those same people endorse the Pill as an alternative to preventing unplanned pregnancies. No unplanned pregnancies, no abortion. Problem solved. Right? Wrong.

What does the Pill have to do with abortion? As this chapter will show, the answer is: Everything.

By the 1960s a huge cultural shift began to take place in America. One of the most profound changes was that sex came out of the bedroom. Studies have shown that between 1965 and 1975 the number of women who had sexual intercourse prior to marriage rose dramatically.[1]

Certainly, there was sexual promiscuity before the '60s. People cheated on their spouses, engaged in premarital sex, and, yes, even had abortions. But those acts were generally frowned upon by society at large. Suddenly, however, behavior that was roundly condemned—including abortion—became the cultural norm.

In the volatile social and political climate of the 1960s, traditional values began to be challenged by a vocal minority. I entered high school in September 1966 and I can remember things changing radically, and fast. In women's fashions, hemlines inched higher while necklines plunged. I distinctly remember TV shows and movies changing. In 1968, I remember the uproar when the movie *Romeo and Juliet* featured a scene with partial nudity. That very brief glimpse of onscreen flesh prompted the Catholic Church to give the film a "B" rating from the Legion of Decency. This "B" rating meant the film was "morally objectionable in part for all." Back in those days, a movie getting a "B" rating meant that Catholics shouldn't see it. (I remember sneaking off with my girlfriends to see the movie, and I know we weren't the only ones.) Television shows, too, began to slip in sexual innuendos. And so society began its journey toward moral decay.

The birth control pill, also born during this decade of upheaval, came about through an unfortunate confluence of science, sociology, and greed. The scientists who developed the Pill were eager to prove they could master the amazingly complex female reproductive system. At the same time, sociologists were busy peddling the dichotomous theories that big families were bad and that everyone should be having a lot of sex. And then there were the pharmaceutical companies that recognized limitless profit when they saw it. It's clear that no one was considering the possibility that the Pill might be bad for women's health, and in fact, more than fifty years later, the health risks of the Pill are still being largely ignored.

On May 10, 1960, the Federal Food and Drug Administration approved the use of the synthetic progesterone pill Enovid as a birth control pill, following a controversial human trial.

Three years before Enovid became the first "Pill," the drug developed by the pharmaceutical company G.D. Searle was given FDA approval for use in treating severe menstrual disorders. The company needed a large-scale human trial to have the drug approved as a contraceptive, so Searle and its scientists, researcher Gregory Pincus, and physician John Rock, looked south to Puerto Rico, a densely populated, impoverished U.S. territory where contraceptives were not illegal. Their quest for a marketable contraceptive was documented in a 2003 film called *The Pill*, which was shown on PBS as part of its "American Experience" series. Even though the producers made no secret of their support for the Pill and the societal changes it wrought, neither did they sugar-coat the contempt the pharmaceutical company and its researchers felt towards their unwitting test subjects. The following paragraphs from the transcript of the series describe the test trials that began in April 1956 in Puerto Rico.

> Dr. Edris Rice-Wray, a faculty member of the Puerto Rico Medical School and medical director of the Puerto Rico Family Planning Association, was in

charge of the trials. After a year of tests, Dr. Rice-Wray reported good news to Pincus. The Pill was 100 percent effective when taken properly. She also informed him that 17 percent of the women in the study complained of nausea, dizziness, headaches, stomach pain and vomiting. So serious and sustained were the reactions that Rice-Wray told Pincus that a 10-milligram dose of Enovid caused "too many side reactions to be generally acceptable."

Rock and Pincus quickly dismissed Rice-Wray's conclusions. Their patients in Boston had experienced far fewer negative reactions, and they believed many of the complaints were psychosomatic. The men also felt that problems such as bloating and nausea were minor compared to the contraceptive benefits of the drug. Although three women died while participating in the trials, no investigation was conducted to see if the Pill had caused the young women's deaths. Confident in the safety of the Pill, Pincus and Rock took no action to assess the root cause of the side effects.

In later years, Pincus's team would be accused of deceit, colonialism and the exploitation of poor women of color. The women had only been told that they were taking a drug that prevented pregnancy, not that this was a clinical trial, that the Pill was experimental or that there was a chance of potentially dangerous side effects.[2]

To this day, questions linger over whether Pincus and Rock, in their rush to bring an effective pill to market, overlooked serious side effects from the high doses of the hormones estrogen and progestin. In fact, when I visited Puerto Rico in 2006 to speak to women's groups in several cities and towns around the island, people shared with me their personal knowledge of the drug trials. Many felt there had been a massive cover-up about the adverse effects on the women who unwittingly participated in this research.

Clearly, the Searle researchers held little regard for women's health. But things must be better now, in this enlightened age of ours, right? Hardly.

While there is ample evidence that the Pill is behind a host of health problems, ranging from some as benign as weight gain to some as serious as fatal blood clots, those who profit from the sale of contraceptives continue to deny that the Pill can harm women. Planned Parenthood is among this group of contraception profiteers, as it has been for decades.

A colleague told me that in 1979 she went to a Planned Parenthood office in her upstate New York college town to get the Pill. She was instructed to take it every evening at 6 p.m. and she remembers vividly that by 11 a.m. the next day, and every day for the ten days she took it, she experienced excruciating ovarian pain and abdominal swelling. When she called Planned Parenthood, they said her problems couldn't possibly be connected to the Pill. She threw them away.

That was thirty years ago, but the medical dangers of the Pill are still widespread. As of July 2012, more than 12,000 personal injury cases had been filed against Bayer Pharmaceutical for its failure to make consumers aware of the health risks of its oral contraceptives Yaz and Yasmin. The company had paid out $402.6 million to settle 1,877 of the suits in the U.S.[3] Plaintiffs suffered pulmonary embolism, heart attack, renal failure, pancreatitis, strokes, and even death. The Yaz and Yasmin contraceptive pills contain drospirenone, a synthetic progestin that has been linked to a greatly increased risk of blood clots. The FDA has ordered the German company to strengthen its blood clot warnings. But why hasn't this pill been recalled? Follow the money: Bayer makes more than $1 billion from Yaz and Yasmin. And don't forget that drug companies are a powerful lobbying force in Washington.

In addition to blood clots[4] the Pill poses numerous, serious health risks to women. Oral contraceptives are indisputably linked to increased risks of cardiovascular disease,[5] cervical and liver cancer,[6] elevated blood pressure,[7] decreased desire and sexual dysfunction,[8] and stroke.[9]

The main health risk question, however, is how the Pill impacts a woman's risk of breast cancer.

The medical community agrees that the risk of breast cancer is greater in women who have an increased exposure to the hormone estrogen. Women who begin menstruating early—before the age of twelve—and experience menopause late—after fifty-five—are at a greater risk of breast cancer because of this extra estrogen. Birth control pills function precisely by increasing a woman's exposure to estrogen. Therefore, the longer a woman takes the Pill, the greater her risk of breast cancer. It seems the argument should end there, but because abortion is such a politically and socially divisive issue, and because contraception and abortion are blood relatives, so to speak, researchers tend to downplay or outright ignore the link between the Pill and an increased risk of breast cancer.

Dr. Angela Lanfranchi, a New Jersey breast cancer surgeon who has been in practice since 1984, said the increased cancer risk is often downplayed by doctors and the media because, statistically, it is a small increase.

"What they neglect to say is that a low risk in millions of women translates into tens of thousands of extra cases of cancer," Dr. Lanfranchi said.

In 1999, combined oral contraceptives (those that use both estrogen and progesterone) were identified as Class 1 carcinogens by the International Agency for Research on Cancer, an arm of the World Health Organization. Following a 2005 review, the designation did not change.[10]

Cancer is not the only problem the Pill causes for women—and society in general. Dr. Lanfranchi pointed to studies showing that oral contraceptives alter a woman's pheromone production and receptivity, and as a result, can cause her to choose the wrong partner for a husband, which could be a contributing factor in our society's high divorce rates.

The *Wall Street Journal* reported on the scientific study that uncovered this pheromone phenomenon in May 2011:

> Much of the attraction between the sexes is chemistry. New studies suggest that when women use hormonal contraceptives, such as birth-control pills,

it disrupts some of these chemical signals, affecting their attractiveness to men and women's own preferences for romantic partners.

The type of man a woman is drawn to is known to change during her monthly cycle—when a woman is fertile, for instance, she might look for a man with more masculine features. Taking the pill or another type of hormonal contraceptive upends this natural dynamic, making less-masculine men seem more attractive, according to a small but growing body of evidence. The findings have led researchers to wonder about the implications for partner choice, relationship quality and even the health of the children produced by these partnerships.[11]

Weird science? Maybe, but even more alarming was the finding of a thirty-nine-year study completed in Great Britain in 2010 that found women who use oral contraceptives are more likely to die a violent death.[12]

*   *   *   *   *

But contraception is one thing, abortion quite another, right?

Wrong.

Even with the advent of the Pill, contraception in the U.S. was only legal for married couples. In 1972, however, the U.S. Supreme Court, ruling in *Eisenstadt v. Baird*, expanded the right of privacy to unmarried people and made contraceptives legally available throughout the country.[13] Just one year later, that same right to privacy would be expanded to include women seeking abortion. For Bill Baird, the named defendant in a Boston case that made its way all the way to the Supreme Court, contraception and abortion go hand in hand.

Even though we are polar opposites on the life issue, Baird and I have been friends for years and he was more than happy to speak with me about his life's work, namely, making contraception and abortion available to poor women. After he saw a woman die following a self-administered abortion in 1963, he worked on the front lines to challenge anti–birth-control laws in New York, New Jersey, and Massachusetts. His *modus operandi* consisted of distributing contraceptives—diaphragms, spermicidal foam, and the Pill among them—until he was arrested. His arrest in front of 2,500 people at Boston University for giving a condom and contraceptive foam to an unmarried woman, became the case that made it to the Supreme Court.

"My goal was to be arrested," he told me. "I arranged to give a condom and a package of contraceptive foam to a nineteen-year-old girl. Twenty cops rushed me and handcuffed me. I also had with me a receipt for $3.09—nine cents was the sales tax—from Zayres Department Store, a big chain in New England, for the Emko foam. I said that if I was being arrested, the attorney general for Massachusetts also should be arrested for collecting sales tax on an illegal item."

Baird was found guilty of a felony in October 1967 and faced up to ten years in prison. His conviction was upheld by the Massachusetts Supreme Court and his first application to bring the case before the U.S. Supreme

Court was rejected. His second appeal was accepted, and on March 22, 1972, the High Court ruled that an individual's right to privacy was paramount to any other consideration. His case, considered by many to be the bedrock on which *Roe v. Wade* was built, is proof that contraception and abortion go hand-in-hand. On that point, Baird and I agree. And the link between the Pill and abortion goes even deeper than these two intimately related court cases.

First, the Pill often acts as an abortifacient. That is, if it fails to prevent conception it will, instead, end conception by not allowing the fertilized egg (a baby) to implant on the uterine wall.

Second, the Pill creates and fosters an abortive mindset. If you're using the Pill, the expectation is that you will not become pregnant. So what if you do? Well, abortion is the next "logical" step. The Pill failed, so now an abortion is needed. The Pill attempts to remove consequences from actions. It attempts to separate cause and effect. It attempts to eliminate children from the act that creates children. And when it fails—or when a woman forgets to take it—the next step is abortion.

*   *   *   *   *

Still not convinced that the Pill is a bad product? Consider its adverse effect on our environment. A 2008 study of male rainbow trout concluded that exposure to estrogen in the environment leads to "diminished reproductive success." You might not be too concerned about rainbow trout, but estrogen excreted in the urine of the millions of women on the Pill is a concern. The study, printed in *The Proceedings of the National Academy of Sciences of the United States of America*, concluded with the following ominous finding:

> Women taking oral contraceptives excrete EE2 (estrogen 17α-ethynylestradiol) and wastewater treatment facilities fail to effectively remove it from the effluent. Thus, increasing levels of the estrogenic contaminant is found in some public water supplies. Levels approaching 8 parts per billion (ppb), or nearly equal to the amount the fish were exposed to in the present study, have been measured in several North American waterways used for irrigation, recreation and drinking. Consequently, male fish are not the only ones exposed or possibly harmed by the findings of this work.[14]

If all the medical and scientific studies aren't enough, let's look logically at the Pill—and what it does. Think about the human body for a moment. Of its many complex systems, the reproductive system—capable of conceiving and sustaining new human life—is the most "wondrously made." It is counterintuitive to accept that if you artificially tinker with this system, for years or even decades, there will be no consequences. Yes, hundreds of millions of women have taken the Pill over the last fifty years and have not developed breast, cervical, or liver cancer, but tens of thousands have been harmed, even killed, by swallowing the lie that avoiding pregnancy is worth any price.

If any other product had caused this much harm to

the American public, even in smaller numbers, wouldn't that product have been recalled?

*   *   *   *   *

The harmful effects of the Pill are well-documented, but what other recourse do women have? What should women do to space out their pregnancies after they throw away their birth control pills? Medical practice regarding regulation of fertility has come a long way and there are methods that are both reliable and consistent with the moral teaching of the Catholic Church. Together these methods are called Natural Family Planning (NFP). In fact, in 2007, a German researcher found NFP to be as reliable as the Pill. Dr. Petra Frank-Hermann, lead author of the report, was quoted in *Science Daily* about her findings.

> For a contraceptive method to be rated as highly efficient as the hormonal pill, there should be less than one pregnancy per 100 women per year when the method is used correctly. The pregnancy rate for women who used the STM (symptothermal method) method correctly in our study was 0.4%, which can be interpreted as one pregnancy occurring per 250 women per year. Therefore, we maintain that the effectiveness of STM is comparable to the effectiveness of modern contraceptive methods such as oral contraceptives, and is an effective and acceptable method of family planning.[15]

It's frankly unbelievable that a safe and natural method

of family planning gets pushed aside for a chemical that causes so much collateral damage.

The Pill also wreaks havoc on women emotionally. Pro-life advocates have long understood that contraception and abortion go hand in hand. Dr. Theresa Burke, co-founder of the post-abortion healing ministry Rachel's Vineyard, discovered the link more than twenty-five years ago in her work:

> I never expected the subject of contraception linked to deep and hidden emotional pain to repeatedly surface during our weekends for healing after abortion. Many abortions are associated with a failure in contraception. Any woman who leaves an abortion clinic is released with an arsenal of birth-control pills. The behavior that led to the pregnancy is never addressed, but she is armed with the resources to prevent another pregnancy . . . or so she thinks. Besides these obvious reasons for grief, I was rather astounded that a growing number of women, including non-Catholics, were coming forward to say that they were also experiencing profound feelings of grief and loss because of contraceptive use which resulted in spontaneous abortions.

I know what Dr. Burke says is true. Years after I stopped taking the Pill, I found myself feeling guilty about the potential lives I snuffed out by my contraceptive habits. I too had profound feelings of grief which I later addressed on a Rachel's Vineyard retreat.

Dr. Peggy Hartshorn, President of Heartbeat International, the first and one of the largest networks of pregnancy help organizations in the world, also noted the link between contraception and abortion years ago when she began helping women with unexpected pregnancies in the mid 1970s. She agrees with Dr. Burke's assertion that many abortions are associated with a failure in contraception.

> I was surprised at first to learn that almost every pregnant girl or woman I worked with had used some form of contraceptive, most often the Pill. Often they stopped because they hated the physical effects such as bloating, loss of libido, weight gain, and worse. Many women then and today express the thought that they did what they had been told is responsible and smart, since they are sexually active, by using the Pill to prevent pregnancy. When they get pregnant anyway, they think it is responsible and smart to have an abortion. This is because they have become convinced that sexual intimacy can and should be separated from child-bearing entirely. Sex for them is recreation—no "creation" is anywhere in their concept of sexual intimacy. Therefore, failures in the Pill lead to abortion—unless these women come in contact with someone, often in a life-affirming pregnancy help center, who can help her capture a new vision of herself as a woman and a new vision of her fertility as a gift, not a problem to be treated with a Pill.

Dr. Hartshorn says she became convinced that women desperately need to learn the truth about their sexuality and this led to Heartbeat's development of the Sexual Integrity program, for use in the over

2,000 pregnancy help centers in the USA. "The truth is that their femininity is based on their physical, emotional, intellectual, and spiritual wholeness as women, a giver and bearer of love and life. Being responsible does not mean taking the Pill or having an abortion. It means respecting oneself and one's God-given dignity as a woman."

And here's another perk for not going down the Pill road. It might save our marriages. Studies have shown that couples who use Natural Family Planning have a much lower rate of divorce than couples who use contraception.[16]

The Pill doesn't deliver on its promises and is clearly detrimental to women. It has clear and well-documented medical side-effects. It damages women psychologically. And it often gets as an abortifacient, while fostering an abortive mindset.

So the next time you think about using the Pill, or recommending it to your teenager daughters, think about all the negatives and ask yourself, is this really empowering women?

CHAPTER ELEVEN

THE GREATEST HOAX

WOMEN NEVER forget their abortions, even if they eventually find healing. Their memories of their abortions become a permanent part of their lives. As we have heard from some of these women in other chapters, not only did abortion not solve their problem, it created many other physical, psychological, and emotional problems.

When I speak at conferences around the country and internationally, women often speak to me about their abortion experience. They have an overwhelming need to have someone understand what abortion did to their lives. Even if they had found healing or forgiveness from a church service or an abortion recovery program there still seemed to be a sense of longing in their voices.

I will never forget the eighty-year-old grandmother who told me: "My abortion was before *Roe v. Wade* made abortion legal and it was not in a back alley as we hear people say, but that abortion haunts me to this day." She said that I was the first person, other than a clergyman, whom she has told about her abortion. She thanked me and confessed, "I regret my abortion." Even at eighty, her decision to have an abortion haunted her.

The abortion industry and the media, however, largely ignore the lasting pain and damage caused by abortion. Planned Parenthood and the other abortion clinics continue their claim of providing simple, safe procedures. They tell women, "Have your abortion today and you can go back to school or work tomorrow." We know that that claim is wildly inaccurate, if not an outright falsehood. The physical pain of abortion is immediate, and it lingers, along with the psychological and emotional scars.

Consider pro-choice politicians (in reality they are pro-abortion), who speak of women's "reproductive health," which is just a sanitized way of saying "the right to kill unborn children." They get their facts, information, and funding from the powerful abortion rights lobbying groups like Planned Parenthood, National Organization for Women, and NARAL Pro-Choice America. Abortion is a billion dollar industry and a powerful lobby in Washington. So where does that leave the women who have bought this product and feel it has failed them? Out in the cold.

In 2002, Georgette Forney and I founded the Silent No More Awareness Campaign with the goal of giving a healing voice to women hurt by abortion and exposing and healing the secrecy and silence surrounding the emotional and physical pain of abortion.

The Campaign began on November 11, 2002. As of July 2012 we have organized 119 gatherings in 10 countries and 48 states, with 5,554 women and men sharing their abortion testimonies. Over 2,600 women and over 300 men have expressed their regret anonymously. There are over 11,750 people, representing 67 countries, registered with the Campaign.

In 2011, we surveyed Campaign members and found that more than half didn't begin looking for healing until after twenty years had passed. People have been conditioned to hide their regret and pain because the culture at large tells us that abortion is just a minor procedure for the benefit of women's health. But women are hurting, deeply, because of abortion.

The stories of these women and men tell the unvarnished truth about abortion.

Steph from Virginia wrote:

> I had an abortion because my parents made me believe there was absolutely no other option for me since I was only 15 years old. I begged until I was exhausted to please allow me to go to an unwed mother's home, deliver the baby and give it up for adoption. NO . . . NO . . . they were not having it! I lived under their roof so I did as they said or else. So, they made the appointment and we left one morning on the three-hour drive. We arrived and I believe (I suppressed these memories so they are still foggy to me) I spoke with the doctor first. He asked me if this was my choice and I said "NO, NOT AT ALL." He said he couldn't do it if it wasn't my choice. He then proceeded to tell me that he was NOT a murderer; if he was, he would be in jail. He also said, that "it" was just a "blob of tissue anyway," as did my parents! He went ahead and did the ultrasound and found out I

was just past my 12-week mark so he told my parents to take me home and give me 48 hours to think about it. Oh man, my stepdad was outside yelling because I didn't do it.

So we went home and they had the entire family coming over, one by one lined up at my bedroom door to come in and tell me that I should have the abortion. Everyone except for my dear Grandmother. She was the only person who stood up for me that whole time. I was so drained by the end of the 48 hours, so exhausted . . . I gave in. I believed that there was no other option.

The abortion was a two-day ordeal. I had to go in one day for the insertion of the seaweed in my cervix to make it dilate. That night, I was having the absolute worst labor-like pains that were actually making me vomit. I kept telling my mom I wanted that medicine out! She did end up calling the doctor and he said if we came back for him to take it out he would just have to reinsert it right away as it had already started the dilation process. I cried and rolled in pain and vomited all night.

When we got back to the clinic the next morning they took me back and gave me Valium. I can remember sitting in a room full of girls as they talked about why they were having their abortion, why it was a bad time for them to be pregnant. There I was, looking to be the youngest in there, waiting in line for my abortion, with tears running down my face. The tears never stopped. During the entire procedure and after when I was in "recovery" I continually cried. I was heartbroken.

Right after, I had recurring nightmares of a baby crying and I would search frantically everywhere and could never find "her!" I've always hated the word abortion and if anyone around me said the word, it made me nauseated. Today, I have some resentment toward my mom and stepdad for putting me through that. I want to ask the both of them . . . did you really think my 12 to 13-week-old fetus was a "blob of tissue" or were you just lying to me? I want to ask them how did they think making that decision for me would affect me 20 years down the road? What gave them the right to put my body and mind through that torture? I thought I had forgiven them years ago but obviously I have not.

Where was Steph's freedom of choice? During a coerced and forced abortion, no one was there to stand up for her rights or the rights of her unborn child!

Daria from Florida wrote:

At age 18 I had a one-year-old son and was in the process of ending an abusive marriage when I became pregnant. I was told everything would be taken care of and was scheduled for an abortion. On that fateful day, I was driven to the abortion clinic and told I would be picked up in a few hours when it was over. Everything in me wanted to run and hide, but I believed there was nowhere to go except inside the clinic. I was frightened and alone as I sat in a room full of strangers, each of us waiting for our name to be called. Once called, I was taken to a small examining room and given a gown to put on. There was absolutely no counseling; no mention of the development of the baby or even that it was anything more than fetal tissue. I was also never told any of the possible side effects of abortion. The doctor came in and without even looking at my face, started the procedure. There was no anesthesia or medication. As I cried out, the nurse's grip on my arms tightened. The sound of the machine seemed deafening, but nothing compared to what I felt inside my womb and heart. After the abortion, they moved me to a recovery room with other women waiting to leave. At the designated time, I walked out of the clinic, feeling completely numb, void of any life.

Within the following year, I fell into deep depression and battled nervous tension that even affected my bodily functions. I developed stomach ulcers and was put on sedatives to which I became addicted. By age 19 I could take no more of the heartache and torment resulting from my abortion and decided one day to end my life (by overdosing on pills). I was found unconscious and rushed to the emergency room, where my stomach was pumped. My life continued, but I lived in hidden shame and guilt, with the pain and knowledge that I was responsible for ending my baby's life. I don't know if there is any greater agony on this earth.

Judy Gonzalez from Florida had the following experience:

When I was a young 17 year old, naïve to the world, I

became pregnant. My parents were devastated, I was confused. Not having a choice, I was whisked away to a New York hospital to have an abortion. As I arrived I remember seeing many, many young and older women there. Some with fear in their eyes, many who didn't seem to care. It was a cold environment, so matter of fact. Next thing I knew I was being prepared and then it was done. As I awoke, I was rushed out of the room to make room for the others. The taxi ride to my aunt's house seemed like an eternity. I had to rest, take the pain medication and returned home to Ohio.

Once home, my whole world took a horrible turn. I did not leave my room for a week, didn't speak with anyone, and didn't do anything but sit and think all day long of what I had done. I had to get to school and back to work so off I went. My guilt was overwhelming; I turned to drugs and promiscuity. I felt I had to punish myself for the horrible thing I had done. This continued for most of my young life. The guilt never left me. I punished myself daily, physically and mentally.

Kimberly Moore from Kentucky wrote:

I was lying on a hospital table in the emergency room. The doctor explained that the abortionist had not completed the procedure and he would need to do a D&C. I didn't even know what that was and I didn't ask. I was too horrified as I faced the realization of what I had buried deep in my heart. I had given permission to someone to kill my child. However, this wasn't the only child I had given someone permission to murder. I'd had two other abortions previously.

The first abortion was when I was in college and my boyfriend and I had just broken up. When I found out several weeks later that I was pregnant, I heard his voice on the other end of the phone saying: "We're too young for this. Our parents will kill us. This wasn't in the plans for my life. I'm continuing my education and can't afford a baby. You can't afford a baby." Feeling embarrassed and thinking my mom would kill me if I came home and told her I was pregnant, and having nowhere else to turn, I agreed to have an abortion. I was pro-choice at the time and had bought into all the lies of my baby just being a conglomeration of cells. But if that were true, why did I feel so bad?

The night after [my first abortion], I went out with my friends and got so drunk I blacked out. I wanted to forget all about what I had done. I continued drinking heavily and almost always blacked out each time I drank. It was the only time I could forget about what I had done. Over time, I started becoming emotionally numb, not caring. I was sinking into depression. My life continued to spiral out of control.

Michele from Kentucky:

I was age 18, life was good. But the spring before I was to leave for college, my birth control failed and I found myself being told by a nurse at a local clinic that I was pregnant. She told me not to worry because I had options. But I already knew which option I would choose. Back then, I not only believed the lie that "it's only a clump of cells," I thought abortion was the most responsible option a young woman in my situation could take. It was the only option that I thought I'd be able to forget once it was done . . . the only option that wouldn't destroy my plans. . . . The only option I thought would affect my life the least. I was selfishly wrong on all three.

The day of my abortion, it seemed like I waited an eternity for my turn with the doctor. I just wanted to get it over with and the longer I laid on that table, the more I started to doubt what I was about to do. A couple of times, I almost got dressed and left. Instead, I kept telling myself what everyone else had told me—that I was doing the right thing . . . and at six weeks it was only cells, right? . . . it wasn't actually a baby yet. . . .

I was wheeled into a room where all I saw was a man wearing a surgical mask at my feet and a nurse standing by my side. During the procedure, I felt a sharp pierce on my left side, heard myself cry out and then it was over. I now know that when my child was severed from my body, even anesthesia couldn't stop the motherly instinct to cry out. It wasn't pain, it was anguish.

But with the same steely determination that had kept me on that table in the clinic, I simply convinced myself to get on with the life I had planned. But I didn't finish college and I didn't marry the father of my child. And though I have accomplished many things, none of them override the value of the life I discarded. You wouldn't know it from the outside, but inside, a part of me was broken; a part of me was missing because my abortion not only left a hole in my womb, it left a huge hole in my heart. And no matter how many ways I tried to fill that hole, it only got deeper.

Connie from Michigan:

At the age of 27, I was a young single mother who had just gotten off welfare and graduated from college. I met a nice young man, who I believed was different from the other men I knew. However, months later when I announced I was pregnant, I wasn't prepared for his response. He told me if I had the baby he would leave me. I was in shock and afraid. Weeks later he made an appointment, drove me to the clinic and paid for the abortion. He went out and waited in the truck. I went inside and spoke with the clinic counselor and told her that I knew that there was life inside my womb and that abortion was against my beliefs, but that my boyfriend coerced me. She didn't discourage me, nor refer me to a local agency for assistance. Ultimately, I made the choice to end my baby's life. From then on I became promiscuous, addicted to alcohol, and prescription drugs. I battled depression and felt hopeless and helpless.

worth and developed bulimia. I hated my parents and rebelled anyway I could.

I have been in therapy since the abortion and within the last couple years I have made a lot of progress. I was caringly persuaded to attend a Rachel's Vineyard retreat in April 2005. This retreat changed my life because although I had always heard 'God forgives you' I never felt it like I did at the retreat. His mercy was falling like rain all around me but I had an umbrella up. The retreat helped me to fold my umbrella and when I did I was drenched in the forgiveness God was pouring out all along. I saw that other women had made the same mistake I did and I didn't condemn them so I realized I needed to stop condemning myself.

People need to know that the babies our country allows to be murdered every day are not lumps of mass, but living children with souls and worth. I felt my baby move inside of me. She had a personality. I left that baby dead in a toilet and my story is multiplied day after day, baby after baby.

It is absurd to think abortion is a solution to any problem. The hurt and pain doesn't end after the baby is gone. I had thought I would just get over it. We are told as women we have a choice, but no one explains what we are choosing. I doubt many would choose to feel the way I have for 10 years so that is why I am Silent No More!"

This is just a small sampling of the testimonies on the Silent No More Awareness Campaign's website.

Women and men come to the site daily, to register their regret for their abortion, and to tell their stories.

Looking at these stories you see many common threads. Symptoms that many women experience after abortion include:

- Bouts of crying
- Eating disorders
- Depression
- Guilt
- Intense grief/sadness
- Anger/rage
- Emotional Numbness
- Lowered self-esteem
- Drug and alcohol abuse
- Flashbacks/Nightmares
- Suicidal urges
- Fear of pregnancy/pregnant women
- Anxiety/panic attacks
- Repeat abortions/crisis pregnancies
- Difficulty with relationships
- Inability to forgive self or others
- Fears of punishment from God

In 2011, Dr. Priscilla Coleman of Bowling Green State University in Ohio released a study in the *British Journal of Psychiatry* that found that women who had an abortion risk facing nearly double the mental health problems as women who have not had an abortion.

Dr. Coleman's study was an analysis of twenty-two earlier studies that looked at the experiences of 877,000 pregnant women, 163,831 of whom had had an abortion.

Coleman wrote:

> Results indicate quite consistently that abortion is associated with moderate to highly increased risks of psychological problems subsequent to the procedure. . . . Overall, the results revealed that women who had undergone an abortion experienced an 81 percent increased risk of mental health problems, and nearly 10 percent of the incidence of mental health problems were shown to be directly attributable to abortion.[1]

Dr. Coleman said abortion leads to greatly increased risk of anxiety disorders, depression, alcohol abuse, and attempted suicide.

Pro-aborts lined up to bash the study as soon as it hit print. The truth is, studies of this type are rarely performed and even more infrequently reported because the abortion lobby wants it that way. But Dr. Coleman's results confirm what post-abortive women have been saying to me for years: abortion hurts women.

Millions of women over the last forty years have bought the product called abortion and, as you have read, this product failed to deliver what it promised.

Isn't it time to recall abortion?

CHAPTER TWELVE

RECALLING A BAD PRODUCT:
A CALL TO ACTION

AFTER ALL the evidence and the testimonies from real women who had real abortions and experienced real pain and suffering, it's clear that abortion is the greatest hoax ever perpetrated upon women.

As such, it's time that we recall abortion.

When a healthy body senses a threat to its well-being, internal or external, it physically responds to repel the threat. When a healthy nation senses a threat to its national security, it responds to repel the threat. These responses are essential to survival.

For our culture to continue to go down the road of abortion-on-demand without even paying attention to, much less trying to avert, the damage abortion is doing, constitutes a failure of our defense systems and raises the question as to whether we have lost the ability to recover. Abortion, along with the blindness to the harm of abortion, places society on a path to self-destruction.

On the other hand, it is a sign of health and a cause for hope if we can muster the strength to both *recall*—to our own minds and to those with whom we communicate—how abortion harms us all, and to *recall* the product which, with false and empty promises, has not only failed to deliver its stated benefits, but has left a path of devastation, the extent of which has only partly been told.

There is a long history of recall in our nation. Products like the Ford Pinto, Firestone tires, Toyota cars, and the Dalkon Shield IUD, just to name a few, were recalled because of the harm they did to some Americans. Abortion's track record is far worse than any of these products.

The abortion procedure itself is the most unregulated medical practice, and it follows none of the standard of care practices found in good medicine. Nail salons have to follow strict regulations covering everything from sanitary practices to technician training, but investigations of clinics where women have died or suffered injury from abortion routinely find filthy conditions and untrained staff. Pets are better protected by the laws regulating veterinary clinics than women are in free-standing abortion clinics.

Consider this: When the American Heart Association discovered that CPR administered quickly to someone having a heart attack could save tens of thousands of lives a year, states began adopting regulations to require schools, restaurants, day care centers, and other businesses to have defibrillators on hand. By 2001, all fifty states had defibrillator laws or regulations on the books. But what we know from former abortion clinic workers and women who have had abortions, as well as investigations into botched abortions, is that these facilities that masquerade as "health care" clinics often don't have this simple life-saving device on hand, nor are clinic personnel trained in its use.

Laurie Wren from Florida worked in an abortion clinic and wrote the following testimony:

> I took a job at the Women's Community Health Center. Since I was a student, I was only available to work two days a week. As it turned out, those were the two days that they did nothing other than perform abortions, from 8 a.m. until 6 p.m.
>
> Looking back I can see the red flags, times I was so uncomfortable, so unsure, signs I should have noticed. But since no one else there seemed adversely affected, I just thought that there must be something wrong with me. After all, the other people working there seemed kind, soft-spoken, considerate. This was my first experience with "the bad guys wearing white." I didn't realize that they were just as deluded as I was.
>
> Often clients would ask me to go with them into the procedure room and hold their hand during their abortion. I remember the sound of that first-trimester suction machine as though it was last week. I remember the young woman with brown hair in the recovery room, who just cried so silently as she stared at the wall. I tried to talk to her; she never heard me. Today I realize that what I know now, she knew then. But I will never forget the day I could no longer deny what was really going on there. Short-handed, a task fell to me that I had never done before. I carried the dark

green trash bag out to the dumpster. I can still feel it across my back to this day! I knew what was inside; they were inside, the aborted babies. I went home, locked my doors, closed all the blinds, unplugged my phone, and lay down on the floor. An overwhelming heaviness seemed to overtake me and hold me there as I asked the question, "Who was in the bag?" Someone with a cure for MS, a president, one of those foster mothers who can love all the hard to love, broken children, someone's best friend, someone's grandson, someone's grandmother! That was just the beginning of a long journey. I had to live through numbing substance abuse, hiding my real self and mountains of shame.

Throughout this book, you have read many of the stories of women who bought this product called abortion hoping it would solve the "problem" of their unexpected pregnancy. But rather than turning back the clock and restoring their former lives, these women found themselves with a new life, full of guilt and recrimination, physical ailments, and emotional darkness. After an abortion, physical problems can include hemorrhage, infection, pelvic inflammatory disease, uterine perforation, hysterectomy, and a compromised cervix which can lead to premature births or miscarriage in future pregnancies. Some women die of their injuries. Psychological problems can include eating disorders, depression, drug and alcohol abuse, and suicidal thoughts. The list goes on and on. No one knows the full extent of the damage abortion does, but the testimonies continue to enlighten us, as do the scientific studies verifying the harmful physical and psychological effects of abortion.

If any product caused just a few of these problems, it would be pulled from the shelves or discontinued as a practice. Yet abortion continues, claiming the lives of more than three thousand children a day in the United States, and forever changing the mothers who made the choice.

If abortion were recalled, it wouldn't be the first time a surgical procedure was halted after proving to be harmful to patients. Bloodletting, for instance, was used for centuries to "cure" all sorts of ailments from pneumonia to back pain.

In the mid-ninteenth century, reputable scientists like Louis Pasteur and Joseph Lister proved that germs caused disease and that bloodletting was a useless procedure. More recently, lobotomies, which were thought to help mental illness, were proved to be phenomenally bad medicine, and they were retired.

The first lobotomies were performed in the 1890s, and by the 1940s and 1950s, the dubious procedure was seen as something of a miracle cure. Tens of thousands of lobotomies were performed in the United States before the procedure fell out of favor in the 1960s for a variety of reasons, including that a growing number of doctors had become skeptical of the operation's therapeutic value.

The transorbital, or "ice pick" lobotomy, was first performed by Dr. Walter Freeman. The doctor used electroshock therapy to render his patient unconscious, then, according to one description, "inserted an ice pick above her eyeball, banged it through her eye socket into her brain and then swirled it around in a sort of egg-beater motion to scramble the neural connections."[1]

This new procedure was seen as a breakthrough because it didn't require opening a patient's skull. As I read about it, I couldn't help thinking about an abortion technique developed by the abortionist Kermit Gosnell (under indictment for murder as this book went to press). His device was a ball of wax with razors inside. Gosnell thought a woman's body temperature would melt the wax and the razors would take care of the baby.

Thinking about lobotomy now, it's hard to imagine how doctors were able to get away with it. Drilling holes through skulls, sometimes pouring alcohol into the brain, flailing around blindly inside the brain with a spatula, jamming ice picks through eye sockets. It's the stuff of science fiction, and yet it happened.

Now think about abortion. In a dismemberment abortion, doctors grope around, often blindly, with their forceps in a woman's uterus until they can grasp a limb of a nearly full-term baby and then proceed to pull it off. Or they insert needles into the heart of a twin in utero, killing him as his or her sibling continues to grow and thrive. Or they send women and girls home with drugs so powerful that their babies are killed and expelled from their wombs in the privacy of their own homes.

Abortion, too, is the stuff of science fiction, and yet it happens thousands of times every day. It was not the first bad product to be unleashed on the American public. Indeed, bad products are recalled all the time. We have laws to protect us from bad products and those laws work. Isn't it time to put consumer protection laws to good use and recall abortion?

*   *   *   *   *

What can we do, practically, to recall abortion?

Here's our plan of action:

1. Sign our on-line petition at www.RecallAbortion. com. We will need a very large number of signatures to present to those who represent us in government. And that's the point: *they represent us*, not the other way around. We govern ourselves, and therefore any concrete legislative plan or judicial strategy that our movement pursues will be stronger when the overwhelming voice of the people echoes and re-echoes their will to be rid of the violence of abortion.

Tell everyone you know about it and urge them to sign it. If they are toeing the pro-choice party line, now is the perfect time to educate them about what abortion really is. Use the information in this book to educate your family, your friends, and your circle of influence. In fact, you might recommend that they read this book together.

2. Spread the stories of the women and men whom have been harmed by abortion, and continue to read the testimonies at www.SilentNoMoreAwareness.org. These individuals have had the courage to speak about the most shameful act of their lives, in order to help others avoid the same pain. Let's match their courage with ours, and for the same motive, by using these testimonies in our own conversations and other communications about abortion.

3. Help people come face to face with their own pain, and find healing. You probably know someone—a sister, niece, cousin, friend, or neighbor—who has had an abortion. You might now be able to recognize the negative effects that abortion had on them. Urge them to find healing through a program like Rachel's Vineyard.

4. Join the Silent No More Awareness Campaign by going to the website and registering. You will receive a monthly E-Letter with news of the Campaign's activities. You don't have to be post-abortive to be Silent No More.

5. One of the most important things you can do is examine the way you think and speak about pregnancy, childbirth, and motherhood. Our culture is anti-life and anti-motherhood. We need to change that, and it starts with each one of us in how we react to pregnancy and the terminology we use.

If you hear that a neighbor's teenage daughter is pregnant, consider your reaction. Do you ask what's she's going to do about it? If you do, you are suggesting that abortion is an option. The better response would be, "How can I help? Is there anything she needs?" Every one of us can play a role in making abortion unthinkable.

A phrase that gets used very frequently is "crisis pregnancy." A more life-affirming description would be "unexpected blessing." No one wishes for a teenage girl to come home with the news that she's pregnant, but it happens. Something as simple as the words we use to react to that news can have a real impact on keeping abortion-vulnerable women away from the killing centers. If we consider babies a blessing, no matter how they were conceived, we begin to give the new mother the emotional support she needs to realize that life is the only choice.

Be aware, also, of how you speak about children. Parents might be asked, "How many children do you have? How many times have you heard the response, "Two and one on the way"? On the way from where? The better response would be, "Two born children and one unborn baby due to be delivered in about four months." Do you see the difference?

When a couple finds out they are expecting a baby, and if they find out the sex of the baby, the best thing to do is to name the baby as soon as possible. I remember when my daughter learned in her fourth month of pregnancy she was carrying a baby girl, she and her husband selected Lily Grace as her name. We began talking to and referring to the baby by her name from that point on. My friend named her unexpected blessing Hope so that when she celebrated her fortieth birthday in her third trimester, she could say "I'm pregnant with Hope."

Why not buy Mother's Day and Father's Day cards for expectant parents? You don't need to wait until the baby is born to count them as mothers and fathers. From the moment of conception they are Moms and Dads, so celebrate it!

Something as simple as the language we use to describe babies and pregnancy can make a difference in bringing about a change in our culture, from pro-abortion to life-affirming.

6. As we work to recall abortion, we must continue

to work on the front lines of the pro-life movement. Become involved in a pregnancy help center in your community (go to www.heartbeatinternational.org to find a list of centers). Devote some time each month to praying outside an abortion facility. Find out how to get in touch with your state and federal representatives and, if they support abortion, become a thorn in their sides. Write letters to newspapers, or comment on online forums when you read a story in the mainstream media that does not tell the truth about abortion. Newspaper websites often give contact information for reporters; contact them directly with your suggestions and constructive criticisms. Get involved with the respect life group at your church, and if there isn't one, organize one!

*   *   *   *   *

This book has repeated the message that it is time to recall abortion. To do so is in fact not only to recall a product, but to *re-call* our government to its proper duty and function, the protection of its citizens. It is to demand that public servants recall their duty to serve the public, not to kill the public. It is to demand that the medical and legal profession recall that at the heart and core of their activity among us is a noble call to serve, shaped by the dignity of the human person. It is, indeed, to recall to action the deepest strength of the human spirit and the character of society which is humble enough to admit when it has been wrong, even when that wrong has been embraced at the most respectable levels of society, and to make course corrections necessary for the common good.

We do this ultimately to insure the well-being of our children and grandchildren, so that the devastation which abortion and its mindset brings may no longer be offered to them under the guise of something that might help resolve their legitimate problems.

Your involvement is vital now to save lives, and it will be just as important once we succeed in recalling abortion. Get involved now because every one of us can make a difference.

You can help bring an end to abortion as an accepted medical procedure.

You can help recall abortion!

REFERENCES

While writing this book, I interviewed many experts who deal with virtually every aspect of abortion—doctors, psychiatrists, and leaders in ministry. I am very grateful for their contributions and I am providing their contact information here so that readers may learn more about their work.

Also, it is with deep gratitude that I thank Georgette Forney with whom I co-founded the Silent No More Awareness Campaign, and the women and men of the Silent No More Awareness Campaign who have, through their own witness, told the truth about this product called abortion. As we say, experience trumps the rhetoric surrounding abortion. Please visit the Campaign website where you can read many, many more of these testimonies. www.SilentNoMoreAwareness.org

John T. Bruchalski, M.D., F.A.C.O.G., OB/GYN
Tepeyac Family Center, LLC; Founder Divine Mercy Care; Chairman www.TepeyacFamily Center.com

Dr. John Bruchalski founded the Tepeyac Family Center in Fairfax, VA in 1994, with the mission of establishing an obstetrical and gynecological facility that combines the best of modern medicine with the healing presence of Jesus

Christ—providing affordable health care to women, in particular, those with crisis pregnancies. In 2000, he founded Divine Mercy Care, a non-profit organization performing spiritual and corporal works of mercy in Northern Virginia, Maryland, and the District of Columbia and is currently the Chairman of its Board of Directors. In 2005, Tepeyac Family Center became a part of Divine Mercy Care and currently operates as the first Catholic healthcare facility in the Diocese of Arlington.

Kevin Burke, MSS/LSW, MEV
Rachel's Vineyard; Executive
Director & Co-Founder
www.RachelsVineyard.org

Kevin Burke is a licensed social worker, Co-Founder of Rachel's Vineyard Ministries, and a Pastoral Associate of Priests for Life. Kevin's presentations address the effects of abortion on men, couples and families. Kevin is the co-author of *Redeeming A Father's Heart-Men Share Powerful Stories of Abortion Loss and Recovery* and *Sharing The Heart of Christ: Safe and Effective Post Abortion Ministry for Clergy and Counselors* co-authored with Dr. Theresa Burke and Fr. Frank Pavone.

Theresa Karminski Burke,
M.A., Ph.D., NCP, LPC, DAPA,
Rachel's Vineyard; Founder
www.RachelsVineyard.org

Theresa Karminski Burke is the founder of Rachel's Vineyard Ministries and the author of *The Rachel's Vineyard Weekend Retreat Manuals* for both Catholic and interdenominational settings. She is also the author of the 15-week support group model *Rachel's Vineyard—A Psychological and Spiritual Journey of Post Abortion Healing* with Barbara Cullen. The Rachel's Vineyard ™ support group and retreat models are now offered in 48 states. The international outreach of Rachel's Vineyard is now growing in 25 countries. Over 700 retreats are held annually world-wide.

Byron Calhoun, M.D., FACOG, FACS CAMC
Family Resource Center
www.camc.org/frc

Dr. Byron C. Calhoun, MD, FACOG, FACS, MBA is a diplomat of the American Board of Obstetrics and Gynecology and is board certified in general Obstetrics/Gynecology and the sub-specialty of Maternal-Fetal Medicine. He has authored 60-plus peer review articles in the obstetric and gynecologic literature, presented more than 100 scientific papers, participated in 40-plus research projects, and published several articles on perinatal hospice. He is an original author of the perinatal hospice concept which provides a multidisciplinary care to families with a lethal prenatal diagnosis. Dr. Calhoun serves as Professor and Vice-Chair in the Department of Obstetrics and Gynecology at West Virginia University-Charleston. He and his wife Kathryn have five children.

Priscilla Coleman, Ph.D. Bowling Green State University School of Family and Consumer Sciences; Human Development and Family Studies; Professor www.bgsu.edu/colleges/edhd/fcs/index.html

Priscilla K. Coleman is a Professor of Human Development and Family Studies at Bowling Green State University in Ohio. She has published articles in peer-reviewed journals suggesting a statistical correlation between abortion and mental health problems, and has claimed in interviews that there is a causal relationship. Coleman's most cited work is "Self-Efficacy and Parenting Quality: Findings and Future Applications", co-authored with Katherine Hildebrandt Karraker in *Developmental Review* Vol. 18, no. 1 (March 1998). She has also published a series of articles reporting a correlation between induced abortion and mental-health problems, findings which have proven controversial.

Mark Crutcher
Life Dynamics; Founder
www.LifeDynamics.com

In 1986, Mark Crutcher committed to working in the pro-life movement full time after years as an outspoken and uncompromised opponent of legalized abortion. At that time, he created the Life Activist Seminar and eventually trained more than 15,000 pro-life activists across the United States and Canada. Then, in 1992, he founded Life Dynamics which has since become widely acknowledged as one of the most innovative and professional pro-life organizations in America.

Mary Davenport, M.D., F.A.C.O.G.
AAPLOG; President
www.aaplog.org

Dr. Mary L. Davenport is current President of the American Association of Pro-Life Obstetricians and Gynecologists (AAPLOG). She is in private practice in the San Francisco Bay area, and lectures widely on abortion complications, medical abortion, world reproductive health, and women's health.

Georgette Forney
Anglicans for Life; President
Silent No More Awareness Campaign; Co-Founder
www.AnglicansForLife.org
www.SilentNoMoreAwareness.org

Georgette Forney is entering her fifteenth year as President of Anglicans for Life, the only global Anglican ministry dedicated to inspiring the Anglican Church to understand and compassionately apply God's Word when addressing abortion, abstinence, adoption, euthanasia, and embryonic stem cell research. She is also the co-founder of the Silent No More Awareness Campaign, an effort to raise awareness about the physical, spiritual, and emotional harm abortion does to women and to let those who are hurting from abortion know help is available. Georgette had an abortion at age sixteen and later experienced healing, forgiveness and reconciliation after going through an abortion recovery program. Through that she developed a greater understanding of the negative impact abortion has on women and the need to highlight the issue as an abortion survivor.

John M. Haas, Ph.D., S.T.L., K.M.
The National Catholic Bioethics Center; President
www.NCBCenter.org

Dr. John M. Haas is the President of The National Catholic Bioethics Center. He received his Ph.D. in Moral Theology from The Catholic University of America and his S.T.L. in Moral Theology from the University of Fribourg, Switzerland. He also has a Master of Divinity degree and has studied at the University of Munich and the University of Chicago

Divinity School. Before assuming the Presidency of The National Catholic Bioethics Center, Dr. Haas was the John Cardinal Krol Professor of Moral Theology at St. Charles Borromeo Seminary of the Archdiocese of Philadelphia and Adjunct Professor at the Pontifical John Paul II Institute for Studies in Marriage and the Family, Washington, D.C.

Margaret Hartshorn, Ph.D.
Heartbeat International; President
www.HeartbeatInternational.org

Margaret H. (Peggy) Hartshorn, answered the call to become involved in the pro-life movement when she heard *Roe v. Wade* announced on the radio, January 22, 1973. Peggy and her husband Mike began housing pregnant women in their home and then established a pregnancy resource center in Columbus, Ohio, opening on January 22, 1981. In 1993, after 20 years as a college English and Humanities professor, Peggy left teaching to lead Heartbeat International, the first life-affirming pregnancy help network founded in the United States and the most expansive in the world (with about 1100 affiliates in 50 countries). It is a Christ-centered association of pregnancy help centers, medical clinics, maternity homes, nonprofit adoption agencies, and abortion recovery programs.

Kristan Hawkins
Students for Life of America; Executive Director
www.StudentsForLife.org

Kristan was hired in 2006 to become Students for Life of America's (SFLA) first Executive Director. Since launching SFLA's full-time operation, Kristan has helped to more than triple the number of campus pro-life groups in the United States, from 181 to over 600, by launching SFLA's Full-Time Field Program. As Executive Director, Kristan directs the mission and strategy of Students for Life of America. Kristan also speaks to youth and adult pro-life organizations across the country to train pro-life activists on how to end abortion in America.

Rebecca Kiessling
Personhood USA; National Spokesperson
www.RebeccaKiessling.com

Rebecca Kiessling is a Family Law attorney, adoptee, home school adoptive mother of five with three biological children and delivers a powerful presentation of her own life story, "Conceived in Rape." Additionally, Rebecca was recently featured in Governor Mike Huckabee's film, "The Gift of Live" and was named national spokesperson for Personhood USA.

As a family law attorney, Rebecca Kiessling litigated numerous high-profile (pro bono) cases, fighting for women's rights as well as the rights of unborn children. She is the "poster child" for Feminists for Life's poster "Did I Deserve the Death Penalty?" and the author of Heritage House '76's pamphlet, "Conceived in Rape: A Story of Hope."

Angela Lanfranchi, M.D., F.A.C.S.
Breast Cancer Prevention Institute; President
www.BCPInstitute.org

Dr. Angela Lanfranchi is a breast cancer surgeon practicing in New Jersey since 1984. She is a member of the Expert Advisory Panel for the New Jersey Board of Medical

Examiners, a member of the Somerset County Cancer Coalition, and on the Professional Advisory Committee of the Wellness Community of Central New Jersey. She is surgical co-director of the sanofi aventis Breast Care Center at the Steeplechase Cancer Center in Somerville, New Jersey. She is co-founder and president of the Breast Cancer Prevention Institute, a non-profit charitable corporation that has as its mission to educate lay and professional communities in the methods of risk reduction and prevention of breast cancer through research, publications and lectures.

Anthony Levatino, M.D., J.D.
Former Abortion Provider

Dr. Anthony Levatino has practiced obstetrics and gynecology since 1980. As a part of his medical training, Dr. Levatino was taught to do abortions. He provided abortions for his patients in his office for eight years. In 1985 he quit doing abortions and is now in private practice as an obstetrician gynecologist.

Troy Newman
Operation Rescue, President
www.OperationRescue.org

Troy Newman has actively worked on behalf of the preborn for over twenty years. Through innovative new tactics, Newman's work is responsible for the closures of dozens of abortion clinics around the nation. He continues as an innovator of new tactics that have helped close abortion clinics and garner criminal prosecutions for abortionists from coast to coast. In 2006, Newman bought and closed Central Women's

Services, an abortion clinic in Wichita, Kansas, that has been renovated and now serves as Operation Rescue's national headquarters and a memorial to the pre-born.

Philip G. Ney, M.D.
International Hope Alive Counselors Association;
Co-Founder
www.Messengers2.com

Raised in Canada, Dr. Ney graduated in medicine from the University of British Columbia and trained as a child psychiatrist and child psychologist at McGill University, London University and the University of Illinois. He is an academic and clinician of over fifty years. He has taught in five medical schools, been full professor three times, served as hospital and academic department chairman, and established three child psychiatric units. He has done research into child abuse for more than forty years and has published many papers and books on this subject. In his early research he became increasingly aware of the connection between child abuse and abortion. Professor Ney has a deep desire to protect children and encourage parents by treating the roots of the problems that make children such vulnerable scapegoats. He lectures in a variety of countries and conducts training seminars in the treatment of Child Abuse and Neglect, Post-Abortion Syndrome, and Post-Abortion Survivor Syndrome.

Anne Nolte, M.D.
Gianna Catholic Healthcare Center for Women, NYC;
Founder and Director
www.SaintPetershcs.com/GiannaCenter

Dr. Anne Nolte (nee Mielnik) is a family physician with an area of concentration in women's health and fertility. She is the Founder and Director of the Gianna Catholic Healthcare Center for Women in New York City, the only women's health center in New York City which offers healthcare for women that is completely in line with Catholic teaching. She has a strong interest in authentic healthcare for women and works to educate women and teenagers about their fertility and reproductive health.

David C. Reardon, Ph.D.
Elliot Institute; Director
www.ElliotInstitute.org

Dr. David C. Reardon director of the Elliot Institute, is widely recognized as one of the leading experts on the aftereffects of abortion on women, a field in which he has specialized since 1983. He is the author of numerous books and popular and scholarly articles on this topic. The emphasis of his work has been on promoting a "pro-woman / pro-life" approach to the abortion issue which emphasizes efforts to prevent coerced and unsafe abortions and efforts to create a more healing environment for women, men and families hurting because of a past abortion.

NOTES

Chapter 2

1. Russell Mokhiber, "Corporate Crime and Violence," *The Multinational Monitor*, April 1987. Volume 8, Number 4. http://multinationalmonitor.org/hyper/ issues/1987/04/editorial.html

Chapter 3

1. Facts on Induced Abortion in the United States, August, 2011, Guttmacher Institute. http://www. guttmacher.org/pubs/fb_induced_abortion.html
2. New York City releases 2010 Abortion Data http:// nyc41percent.com/
3. Facts on Induced Abortion in the United States, August 2011, Guttmacher Institute. http://www. guttmacher.org/pubs/fb_induced_abortion.html
4. Investigation of Women's Medical Society by the Office of the District Attorney, City of Philadelphia http://www.phila.gov/districtattorney/grandjury_ womensmedical.html

5. "Operator of Clinics is Charged," *Los Angeles Times*, February 2008 http://articles.latimes.com/2008/feb/08/local/me-abortion8

6. Background check on Pierre Renelique http://www.healthgrades.com/physician/dr-pierre-renelique-ypt4p/background-check

7. "$1.9M settlement in botched abortion," NorthJersey.com, December 2009 http://www.northjersey.com/news/19M_settlement_in_botched_abortion.html?c=y&page=2

8. "Pro-choice co-founder rips abortion industry," *World Net Daily*, December 2002 http://www.wnd.com/2002/12/16344

Chapter 4

1. "Did Abortion Legalization Reduce the Number of Unwanted Children?" Evidence from Adoption, Guttmacher Institute, Jan.-Feb. 2002 http://www.guttmacher.org/pubs/journals/3402502.html

2. State of America's Children 2010 Report, Children's Defense Fund, May 2010. http://www.childrensdefense.org/child-research-data-publications/data/state-of-americas-children-2010-report.html

3. Estimated Age at First Marriage, By Sex, 1890 to 2010. www.census.gov/population/socdemo/hh-fam/ms2.xls

4. *Instruction on Respect for Human Life* can be found at http://www.vatican.va/roman_curia/congreations/

cfaith/documents/rc_con_cfaith_doc_19870222_
respect_for_human_life_en.html
Dignitatis Personae can be found at: http://www.
vatican.va/roman_curia/congregations/cfaith/
documents/re_con_cfaith_doc_20081208_
dignitatis_personae_en.html

5. "The Two Minus One Pregnancy," *New York Times Magazine*, August 2011 http://www.nytimes.com/2011/08/14/magazine/the-two-minus-one-pregnancy.html?pagewanted=all

6. Umberto Castiello, et al. "Wired To Be Social: The Ontogeny of Human Interaction," Plos One 5 (10) October 2010. http://www.plosone.org/article/info%3Adoi%2F10.1371%2Fjournal.pone.0013199

Chapter 5

1. Susan B. Anthony, quoted in Frances Willard's *Glimpses of Fifty Years: The Autobiography of an American Woman*. Chicago: Women's Temperance Pub. Assoc., 1889, 598

2. Ashley Herzog, *Feminism Vs. Women*, Xulon Press, 2008, 87.

3. The Public Writings and Speeches of Margaret Sanger, 1911-1960. http://www.nyu.edu/projects/sanger/webedition/app/documents/show.php?sangerDoc=236637.xml

4. Live Action blog, http://liveaction.org/blog/planned-parenthood-1952-abortion-kills-baby/

5. National Health Statistics Reports, Number 49,

March 22, 2012, Page 9 http://www.cdc.gov/nchs/data/nhsr/nhsr049.pdf

Chapter 6

1. Guttmacher Institute, Facts on Induced Abortion in the U.S. August 2011 http://www.guttmacher.org/pubs/fb_induced_abortion.html

2. Gonzales, Attorney General, v. Carhart et al., April 18, 2007, 3a http://caselaw.lp.findlaw.com/scripts/getcase.pl?court=US&vol=000&invol=05-380&friend=nytimes

Chapter 7

1. *Victims and Victors: Speaking Out About their Pregnancies, Abortions and Children Conceived in Sexual Assault.* Edited by David C. Reardon, Julie Makimaa, and Amy Sobie. Dover, DE: Acorn, Acorn Books, 2000.

2. Shauna R. Prewitt, "Giving Birth to a 'Rapist's Child': A Discussion and Analysis of the Limited Legal Protection Afforded to Women Who Become Mothers Through Rape." *Georgetown Law Journal*, Volume 100, Issue 3, Pages 827-862.

3. Guttmacher Institute, State Policies in Brief as of November 1, 2012. "Abortion Reporting Requirements" http://guttmacher.org/statecenter/spibs/spib_ARR.pdf

4. Felicia H. Stewart and James Trussel, "Prevention of Pregnancy Resulting from Rape," *American Journal of*

Preventive Medicine, Volume 19, Issue 4, November 2000, 228-229. http://www.ajpmonline.org/article/ S0749-3797(00)00243-9/abstract

5. Melissa Holmes, Heidi Resnick, Dean Kilpatrick, and Connie Best, "Rape-Related Pregnancy: Estimates and Descriptive Characteristics from a National Sample of Women," *American Journal of Obstetrics and Gynecology*, Volume 175, Issue 2, August 1996, 32-325. http://www.ajog.org/article/ S0002-9378(96)70141-2/abstract

6. Lawrence B. Finer, et. al., "Reasons U.S. Women Have Abortions: Quantitative and Qualitative Perspectives," *Perspectives on Sexual and Reproductive Health*, Volume 37, Number 3, 2005. http://www. guttmacher.org/pubs/journals/3711005.pdf

Chapter 8

1. American College of Obstetricians and Gynecologists (ACOG). "ACOG Statement of Policy: ACOG Policy on Abortion." January 1993

2. "The Limits of Conscientious Refusal in Reproductive Medicine," American College of Obstetricians and Gynecologists Committee Opinion. Number 385. November 2007. http://www.acog.org/ Resources_And_Publications/Committee_ Opinions/Committee_on_Ethics/The_Limits_of_ Conscientious_Refusal_in_Reproductive_Medicine

3. Brady Begeal, "Burdened by Life: A Brief Comment on Wrongful Birth and Wrongful Life." *Albany*

Government Law Review. Volume 4, 870-876. March 28, 2011. http://www.albanygovernmentlaw-review.org/files/Begeal_2_Pro_Format_NEW.pdf

4. Bethanne Scholl, "Colby's Story." *The Leaven*, October 2002. http://www.theleaven.com/oldleavenwebsite/archives/oct02.html

Chapter 9

1. What is AAPLOG's Position on "Abortion to Save the Life of the Mother?" July 2009. http://www.aaplog.org/position-and-papers/abortion-to-save-the-life-of-the-mother/

2. Emily Allen, "Cancer mother who refused to abort her baby for the sake of her own health now in remission and has a healthy little girl." *Daily Mail*, August 1, 2012. http://www.dailymail.co.uk/health/article-2182041/Cancer-mother-refused-abort-baby-sake-health-remission-healthy-little-girl.html

3. Peter Baklinski, "A Thanksgiving gift: mother with aggressive cancer gives birth to healthy baby despite treatment," LifeSiteNews.com November 17, 2011. http://www.lifesitenews.com/news/a-thanksgiving-gift-mother-with-aggressive-cancer-gives-birth-to-healthy-ba/

4. Thomas Murphy Goodwin, "Medicalizing Abortion Decisions." *First Things*. March 1996. http://www.firstthings.com/article/2007/10/003-medicalizing-abortion-decisions-15

5. "Ectopic for Discussion: A Catholic Approach to Tubal Pregnancies." Catholics United for the Faith, 2004. http://www.cuf.org/faithfacts/details_view.asp?ffID=57

Chapter 10

1. Heer; Amyra Grossbard-Shechtman, "The Impact of the Female Marriage Squeeze and the Contraceptive Revolution on Sex Roles and the Women's Liberation Movement in the United States, 1960 to 1975," *Journal of Marriage and the Family*, Vol. 43, No. 1. (Feb., 1981), pp. 49-65).

2. Excerpts from transcript of *The Pill*, produced and directed by Chana Gazit, 2003, aired on PBS "American Experience" series. http://www.pbs.org/wgbh/amex/pill/filmmore/fd.html

3. "Bayer's Yasmin Lawsuit Settlements Rise to $402.6 Million." *Bloomberg News*. July 31, 2012. http://www.businessweek.com/news/2012-07-31/bayer-s-yasmin-lawsuit-settlements-rise-to-402-dot-6-million

4. FDA Drug Safety Communication: Updated information about the FDA-funded study on risk of blood clots in women taking birth control pills containing drospirenone, Updated October 2011 http://www.fda.gov/Drugs/DrugSafety/ucm277346.htm

5. Shufelt, Baire Merz, "Contraceptive Hormone Use and Cardiovascular Disease," *Journal of the American College of Cardiology*, Jan. 20, 2009. http://content.onlinejacc.org/cgi/content/full/53/3/221?maxtoshow=&hits=10&RESULTFORMAT=&fulltext=contraception+shufelt+mertz&searchid=1&FIRSTINDEX=0&resourcetype=HWCIT

6. National Cancer Institute "Fact Sheet," reviewed 5/04/06 http://www.cancer.gov/cancertopics/factsheet/Risk/oral-contraceptives

7. American Heart Association, "High Blood Pressure and Women," Updated February 2012 http://www.heart.org/HEARTORG/Conditions/HighBloodPressure/UnderstandYourRiskforHighBloodPressure/High-Blood-Pressure-and-Women_UCM_301867_Article.jsp

8. Wallwiener, Wallwiener, Seeger, Mück, Bitzer, Wallwiener, "Prevalence of Sexual Dysfunction and Impact of Contraception in Female German Medical Students," *Journal of Sexual Medicine*, Volume 7, Issue 6, pages 2139–2148, June 2010 http://onlinelibrary.wiley.com/doi/10.1111/j.1743-6109.2010.01742.x/full

9. American Heart Association/American Stroke Association, "Hidden Risk Factors for Women," Updated January 2011 http://www.strokeas sociation.org/STROKEORG/AboutStroke/ UnderstandingRisk/Hidden-Risk-Factors-for-Women_UCM_310403_Article.jsp

10. World Health Organization, Carcinogenicity of combined hormonal contraceptives and combined menopausal treatment, September 2005 http:// www.who.int/reproductivehealth/topics/ageing/ cocs_hrt_statement.pdf

11. Alvergne, Alexandra and Lummaa, Virpi, "Does the Contraceptive Pill Alter Mate Choice in Humans," *Trends in Ecology & Evolution*, March 2010 http://www.sciencedirect.com/science/article/ pii/S0169534709002638 http://online.wsj.com/article/SB100014240527487 04681904576313243579677316.html

12. Hannaford, Iversen, Macfarlane, Elliott, Angus and Lee, "Mortality among contraceptive pill users: cohort evidence from Royal College of General Practitioners' Oral Contraception Study," *British Medical Journal*, March 11, 2010. http://www.ncbi. nlm.nih.gov/pmc/articles/PMC2837145/

13. *Eisenstadt v. Baird*, 405 US 438 (1972) http:// caselaw.lp.findlaw.com/cgi-bin/getcase. pl?court=us&vol=405&invol=438

14. Brown, Schultz, Cloud, Nagler, "Aneuploid sperm formation in rainbow trout exposed to the environmental estrogen 17α-ethynylestradiol," Proceedings of the National Academy of Sciences of the United States of America, Dec. 9, 2008 http://www.pnas.org/content/105/50/19786

15. European Society for Human Reproduction and Embryology (2007, February 21). Natural Family Planning Method As Effective As Contraceptive http://www.sciencedaily.com/releases/2007/02/070221065200.htm

16. Arzu Wilson, "The Practice of Natural Family Planning Versus the Use of Artificial Birth Control: Family, Sexual and Moral Issues," *Catholic Social Science Review*, Vol VII, Nov. 2002 http://cssronline.org/CSSR/

Chapter 11

1. Priscilla K. Coleman, "Abortion and mental health: quantitative synthesis and analysis of research published 1995-2009." *British Journal of Psychiatry*, Volume 199, Pages 180-186. September 2011. http://bjp.rcpsych.org/content/199/3/180

Chapter 12

1. "My Lobotomy." Sound Portraits Productions, 2005. http://soundportraits.org/on-air/my_lobotomy/

ACKNOWLEDGMENTS

This book would never have come to fruition had it not been for the inspiration of the Holy Spirit. To the Disciples of the Lord Jesus Christ, in Prayertown, TX—thank you, Sisters, for your prayers and encouragement. Fr. Frank Pavone—thank you for your spiritual direction, for believing in me and setting me on deadlines to get the ideas in my head onto paper. Anthony DeStefano—thank you for your expertise in the publishing industry, for keeping me on track, and for being such a great friend over these three decades. Leslie Palma-Simoncek, my research assistant—thank you for ALL you did to help me make this book a reality. Peter Miller—thank you for being such a great literary manager. And finally, to Christian Tappe, my editor, and all the other wonderful folks at Saint Benedict Press—thank you for publishing this book and for doing it in record time!

ABOUT THE AUTHOR

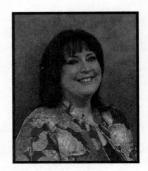

JANET MORANA is Executive Director of Priests for Life and Co-Founder of the Silent No More Awareness Campaign (www.silentnomoreawareness.org), the world's largest mobilization of women who have had abortions.

Born in Brooklyn, NY, she holds a Master's degree in Education and was a full-time public school teacher.

She is a national pro-life leader and assists the Vatican on pro-life matters.

She co-hosts the *Defending Life* and *The Catholic View for Women* series on EWTN, and is a frequent guest on other TV and radio programs. In 2003, she addressed the Pro-Life Caucus of the U.S. House of Representatives on life issues. She is the recipient of Legatus' Cardinal John O'Connor Pro-life Hall of Fame Award.

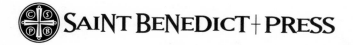
SAINT BENEDICT † PRESS

Saint Benedict Press publishes books, Bibles, and multimedia that explore and defend the Catholic intellectual tradition. Our mission is to present the truths of the Catholic faith in an attractive and accessible manner.

Founded in 2006, our name pays homage to the guiding influence of the Rule of Saint Benedict and the Benedictine monks of Belmont Abbey, just a short distance from our headquarters in Charlotte, NC.

Saint Benedict Press publishes under several imprints. Our TAN Books imprint (TANBooks.com), publishes over 500 titles in theology, spirituality, devotions, Church doctrine, history, and the Lives of the Saints. Our Catholic Courses imprint (CatholicCourses.com) publishes audio and video lectures from the world's best professors in Theology, Philosophy, Scripture, Literature and more.

For a free catalog, visit us online at
SaintBenedictPress.com

Or call us toll-free at
(800) 437-5876

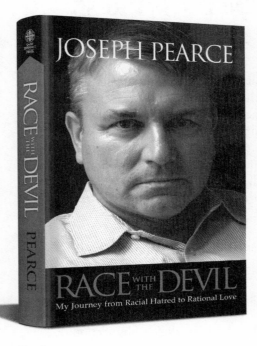

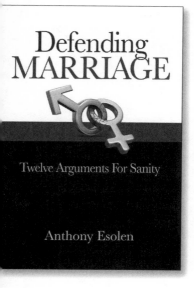
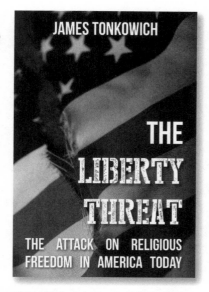